PEDIATRIC NCLEX-RN REVIEW:

200 Practice Questions with Detailed Rationales Explaining Correct and Incorrect Answer Choices

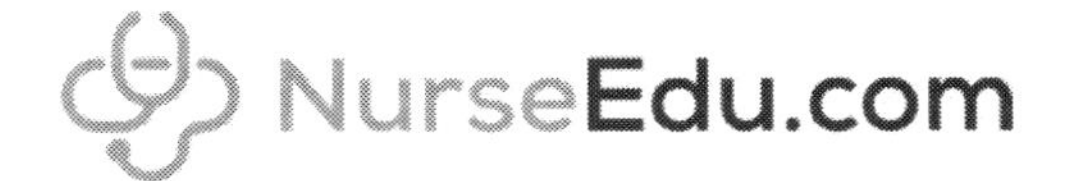

Disclaimer:

Although the author and publisher have made every effort to ensure that the information in this book was correct at press time, the author and publisher do not assume and hereby disclaim any liability to any party for any loss, damage, or disruption caused by errors or omissions, whether such errors or omissions result from negligence, accident, or any other cause.

This book is not intended as a substitute for the medical advice of physicians. The reader should regularly consult a physician in matters relating to their health and particularly with respect to any symptoms that may require diagnosis or medical attention.

NCLEX®, NCLEX®-RN, and NCLEX®-PN are registered trademarks of the National Council of State Boards of Nursing, Inc. They hold no affiliation with this product.

Some images within this book are either royalty-free images, used under license from their respective copyright holders, or images that are in the public domain.

For bulk orders or questions, reach out to Support@NurseEdu.com

ISBN: 978-1-952914-15-7

FREE BONUS

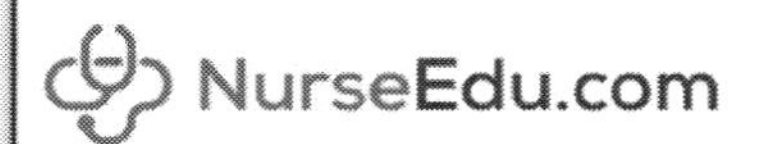

Mnemonics
LAB VALUES
CHEATSHEET

Explore Mnemonics Used in Nursing School & Most Commonly Found on The NCLEX.

FREE Download – Just Visit:

NurseEdu.com/bonus

TABLE OF CONTENTS:

CHAPTER 1:

NCLEX-RN – PEDIATRIC: EENT - 25 QUESTIONS

1. The recovery room nurse is caring for a 9-year-old girl who is recovering from tonsillectomy. The child is sleepy but easily awakened. The nurse knows the child should be placed in which position?

   A. Supine
   B. Side-lying
   C. Prone
   D. Sims'

Rationale:

Correct answer: B

Tonsillectomy is an outpatient procedure performed to remove the tonsils due to recurrent tonsillitis, airway obstruction, or debris (tonsil stones). The patient is at risk for bleeding in the throat immediately following the surgery, so keeping the airway patent and facilitating oral drainage is most important. Side-lying is the best position to place the child. The nurse should frequently monitor vital signs, watching especially for decreasing blood pressure and increasing heartrate. Bright red blood in the back of the throat is another sign of hemorrhage.

A is incorrect because if the patient experiences bleeding in the throat, supine position could lead to bleeding into the airway.

C is incorrect because prone position is inappropriate as it does not facilitate easy breathing after surgery.

D is incorrect because Sims' position is for administration of an enema.

2. The nurse in the clinic is preparing to instill antibiotic eyedrops in a 12-year-old boy with bacterial conjunctivitis. In order to avoid systemic adverse effects from the medication, which of the following does the nurse perform?

    A. Apply pressure on the eyelid rim
    B. Apply pressure on the inner canthus
    C. Place the child supine after instillation
    D. Have the child close their eyes tightly

Rationale:

Correct answer: B

Conjunctivitis, or pinkeye, is erythema and swelling of conjunctiva due to infection with a virus or bacteria and is highly contagious. Only bacterial conjunctivitis is treated with antibiotic eye drops. After the eyedrops are instilled, the child closes their eyes gently, and light pressure is applied to the inner canthus for a couple of minutes to prevent the medication from being absorbed systemically.

A is incorrect because applying pressure on the eyelid rim will not prevent systemic absorption. This will prevent the medication from washing over the surface of the eye and prevent the full effect of the medication.

C is incorrect because placing the child supine will not prevent systemic absorption but may cause the eyedrops to leak out of the lateral surfaces of the eyes.

D is incorrect because having the child close their eyes tightly will cause the eyedrops to be expressed from the eyes and run down the cheeks. This will prevent the medication from having the desired antibacterial effect on the infected eyes.

3. The nurse in the clinic is caring for a 7-year-old girl experiencing epistaxis. The nurse performs which of the following interventions?

   A. Performs abdominal thrust maneuver (Heimlich)
   B. Applies ice collar to neck
   C. Compresses nares to septum for at least 5 minutes
   D. Encourages throat gargles with warm saline

Rationale:

Correct answer: C

Epistaxis is a nosebleed and can either be anterior or posterior, depending on where mucosa has been eroded and blood vessels are exposed. Compressing the nares to the septum for at least 5 minutes places pressure on the exposed blood vessel and stops bleeding.

A is incorrect because the Heimlich maneuver is for foreign object removal from the airway and may worsen epistaxis.

B is incorrect because an ice collar applied to the neck will not relieve epistaxis.

D is incorrect because throat gargles with warm saline are appropriate after epistaxis is resolved but will not relieve epistaxis and are, therefore, not the best nursing action.

4. A 5-year-old boy is in the clinic complaining of ear pain. When assessing the child, which of the following findings would alert the nurse to consider serous otitis media?

A. Inflammation of the external ear and crust on the auditory canal
B. Sensorineural hearing loss and tinnitus
C. Plugged feeling in ear and reverberation of child's own voice
D. Tympanic membrane is bright red and bulging or retracted and fever

Rationale:

Correct answer: C

Serous otitis media occurs when the eustachian tube is blocked from a nasal allergy attack or upper respiratory infection, causing fluid collection in the middle ear. The child will experience a plugged feeling in the ear and hear their own voice reverberating due to the fluid collection.

A is incorrect because inflammation of the external ear is otitis externa.

B is incorrect because sensorineural hearing loss and tinnitus are due to inner ear damage, which can be a long-term detrimental result from untreated otitis media.

D is incorrect because an inflamed tympanic membrane with fever is myringitis.

5. A 9-year-old girl in the clinic has been diagnosed with strep throat. When assessing the child, which findings does the clinic nurse expect to find?

A. Weak cough and high-pitched noise with respirations
B. Foul breath and noisy respirations
C. Pain over sinus areas and purulent nasal secretions
D. Bright red pharynx and fever

Rationale:

Correct answer: D

Strep throat is a bacterial streptococcal infection of the throat. The throat becomes bright red and raw with or without white or yellow spots, and the child will complain of pain when swallowing. Tonsils and lymph nodes become swollen, and the child will have a fever with this diagnosis.

A is incorrect because strep throat does not cause a weak cough or high-pitched noise with respiration. Weak cough may be an indication of a child who is lethargic or has impaired respiratory muscles, and high-pitched noises may indicate narrowing of the airways, which is not common with strep throat.

B is incorrect because strep throat may cause foul breath but does not commonly cause noisy respirations. Noisy respirations can be an indication of croup (presents with inspiratory stridor) or constricted airway channels and should be investigated further by the nurse.

C is incorrect because strep throat does not cause sinus pain or purulent nasal secretions. These are symptoms of a sinus infection.

6. A 5-year-old female child is in the emergency room for an item lodged in the left ear. The parent states that it may be a mosquito. Which of the following nursing actions is best?

  A. Irrigation of the ear with warm water
  B. Instillation of diluted alcohol
  C. Instillation of antibiotic ear drops
  D. Instillation of corticosteroid ear drops

Rationale:

Correct answer: B

Insects in the ear are typically killed with instillation of diluted alcohol unless a flashlight or humming noise coaxes them out. The diluted alcohol is instilled to suffocate the insect, which can then be removed from the ear with forceps.

A is incorrect because irrigation of the ear with water can be detrimental to the child if the object is a piece of food (beans, seeds, and small vegetables will swell with water irrigation, making them more difficult to remove from the ear). If the nurse visualizes an insect in the ear, water, mineral oil, or alcohol can be instilled to suffocate the insect.

C is incorrect because antibiotic ear drops will not remove an insect and are not necessary unless signs of infection are present. The insect would be removed from the ear first (with oil or alcohol), and then the infection can be treated.

D is incorrect because corticosteroid ear drops will not remove an insect and are usually not necessary. (It is important for the nurse to use non-pharmacologic measures when possible.)

7. A 7-year-old boy is in the clinic complaining of ear pain. The nurse questions orders for ear canal irrigation in which of the following circumstances?

   A. Wax buildup
   B. Hearing loss
   C. Otitis externa
   D. Perforated tympanic membrane

Rationale:

Correct answer: D

Irrigation of the ear canal when the tympanic membrane is perforated is contraindicated as fluid can enter the inner ear, causing dizziness, infection, nausea, and vomiting.

A is incorrect because ear pain could be due to cerumen impaction, which may be irrigated.

B is incorrect because hearing loss could be due to cerumen impaction, which may be irrigated.

C is incorrect because otitis externa is due to either infection or cerumen impaction, which may be irrigated.

8. The school nurse is preparing to perform a hearing assessment on a 10-year-old girl. When performing the whispered voice test, which of the following is the correct method for performing the test?

   A. Stand 4 feet away from the child to ensure the child can hear from this distance.
   B. Stand 1-2 feet in front of the child, whisper, a statement and have the child repeat it.
   C. Whisper a statement with the nurse's back facing the child.
   D. Stand 1-2 feet behind the patient, have the child plug one ear, whisper three letters or numbers, and have the child repeat the sequence.

Rationale:

Correct answer: D

This is the proper method for performing the voice hearing assessment. The process is then repeated using a different letter or number sequence with the patient's other ear blocked.

A is incorrect because standing 4 feet away is not the correct distance for performing the voice hearing assessment.

B is incorrect because standing in front of the child does not prevent lip-reading.

C is incorrect because the nurse's back should not be facing the child. The nurse should stand 1-2 feet behind the patient, facing the patient's back.

9. The nurse has received orders for instillation of cortisporin suspension, 2 gtts right ear, for an 8-year-old boy in the clinic. Which of the following interventions is essential for the nurse to perform?

   A. Verify correct patient and route
   B. Warm the solution before instilling, to prevent dizziness
   C. Hold an emesis basin under the child's ear
   D. Position the child in semi-Fowler's

Rationale:

Correct answer: A

The nurse always follows the five rights of medication administration, which begins with verifying the correct patient and route. Two forms of patient identifier must be used.

B is incorrect because the solution may be instilled at room temperature.

C is incorrect because an emesis basin under the ear is used for irrigation. When administering 2 gtts into the ear, the nurse would not anticipate anything to drain out of the ear.

D is incorrect because the child should be placed in a side-lying position, not semi-Fowler's.

10. The nurse in the clinic is assessing a 12-month-old child with cleft palate who is awaiting surgical repair in 2 weeks. The nurse knows the child is at increased risk for otitis media due to:

    A. Lowered resistance to infection due to decreased nutritional intake
    B. Dysfunction of eustachian tubes
    C. Eustachian tube plugging with food particles
    D. Middle ear congenital defects

Rationale:

Correct answer: B

Cleft palate is a congenital defect that affects the palate, or roof of mouth, and prevents tissue from completely closing in utero, leaving an opening between the roof of the mouth and the nasal passage. The eustachian tubes may also be dysfunctional or ineffective due to the structural defect, putting the child at increased risk for otitis media. Cleft palate is often repaired between the ages of 12 and 18 months.

A is incorrect because children with cleft palate do not necessarily have altered nutrition. Parents should be taught that these babies often take longer to feed and need adequate time to finish meals. Soft nipple may be needed for bottle-feeding, and they should be burped often.

C is incorrect because food does not commonly enter the eustachian tube through the cleft palate.

D is incorrect because cleft palate and congenital middle ear deformities are not associated.

11. The nurse in the newborn nursery is assessing an infant who has a cleft lip. Which of the following nursing actions is best?

   A. Assessing sucking ability
   B. Monitoring for adequate diaphragmatic movement
   C. Encouraging locomotion
   D. Administering ranitidine to promote GI function

Rationale:

Correct answer: A

Cleft lip is a congenital defect that affects the upper lip and prevents tissue from completely joining in utero, leaving a separated upper lip that may affect the nose as well. Assessing sucking ability is the nurse's greatest priority as it directly impacts the infant's nutritional needs. The infant will have difficulty with sucking, and devices may be required to allow the infant to feed adequately and be gratified by sucking.

B is incorrect because cleft lip does not affect movement of the diaphragm. Respiratory status should be monitored closely, however, especially during feeding, when the infant is more at risk for aspiration.

C is incorrect because cleft lip does not affect locomotion. The primary concern is ability to suck and swallow and maintain airway during feedings. This is more important than mobility.

D is incorrect because cleft lip does not primarily affect GI function. Ranitidine is not routinely given to infants with cleft lip unless reflux is present.

12. The nurse in the recovery room is caring for a 5-year-old boy who just underwent tonsillectomy. When observing the boy, which of the following would the nurse report to the surgeon immediately?

    A. Vomiting episode
    B. Blood trickling down the throat
    C. Dark brown blood on teeth
    D. Complains of sore throat

Rationale:

Correct answer: B

Tonsillectomy is an outpatient procedure performed to remove the tonsils due to recurrent tonsillitis, airway obstruction, or debris (tonsil stones). Blood trickling down the throat indicates bleeding is occurring from the surgical site and warrants immediate notification of the surgeon.

A is incorrect because vomiting commonly occurs after surgery and does not need to be reported. The nurse should be prepared to administer antiemetics, keep the patient NPO, and position the patient to prevent aspiration of vomitus.

C is incorrect because dark brown blood on the teeth is "old blood" and does not need to be reported. Bright red blood is an indication of current bleeding, which is the priority concern.

D is incorrect because a sore throat is expected after tonsillectomy and does not need to be reported to the healthcare provider.

13. The nurse is assessing a 5-month-old infant girl with oral candidiasis. Which of the following related conditions does the nurse assess the infant for?

    A. Aphthous ulcers
    B. Herpes simplex infection
    C. Diaper rash
    D. Eczema

Rationale:

Correct answer: C

Oral candidiasis, or thrush, is a yeast or candida infection in the mouth. The infection can spread through the GI tract to the anus and can also spread as a result of poor hand hygiene performed by the nurse or caregiver. Diaper rash is a common finding with oral candidiasis.

A is incorrect because aphthous ulcers (commonly called canker sores) are not related to oral candidiasis. Often, the cause of aphthous ulcers is unknown. They last 10 to 14 days, usually heal without the need for medication, and don't commonly leave a scar.

B is incorrect because herpes simplex infection is caused by the herpes simplex virus and is not related to oral candidiasis.

D is incorrect because eczema is a group of skin conditions (skin becomes inflamed and irritated) that are not related to oral candidiasis.

14. A 4-year-old boy who has experienced frequent ear infections is diagnosed as having mixed hearing loss. Which of the following complications does the clinic nurse assess the boy for?

    A. Recurring temporal headaches
    B. Mandible inflammation
    C. Delayed language development
    D. Serosanguineous ear drainage

Rationale:

Correct answer: C

Mixed hearing loss is due to damage to both the inner ear and the middle or outer ear, and is a combination of sensorineural as well as conductive hearing loss. Children who experience hearing loss, regardless of the cause, are at increased risk for delayed language development. Children learn to speak by listening and replicating sounds, and if hearing is damaged, then speech cannot be replicated.

A is incorrect because recurring temporal headaches are unrelated to mixed hearing loss. Muscle injury, inflammation, or viral infection are more commonly the cause of recurring temporal headaches.

B is incorrect because mandible inflammation is unrelated to mixed hearing loss.

D is incorrect because sero-sanguineous ear drainage is due to infection or trauma to the inner or middle ear.

15. The nurse in the emergency room has just admitted a 4-year-old boy whose temperature is 104°F (40°C) and has inspiratory stridor, restlessness, and is leaning forward and drooling. What is the nurse's priority?

    A. Auscultate lungs and place the boy in a CO_2 mist tent
    B. Encourage PO fluids and reduce anxiety
    C. Examine the boy's throat and perform throat culture
    D. Notify the healthcare provider immediately and prepare for intubation

Rationale:

Correct answer: D

This child has classic signs of acute epiglottitis, or inflammation of the epiglottis. This is an airway emergency in pediatric patients. The nurse must notify the healthcare provider immediately and prepare for intubation.

A is incorrect because the nurse already knows the boy is experiencing inspiratory stridor and exhibiting signs of respiratory distress. A CO_2 mist tent will not help relieve epiglottitis. The boy needs humidified oxygen and potentially intubation.

B is incorrect because PO fluids are not safe for a patient in respiratory distress. IV fluids should be administered. Anxiety reduction is important, but this is a psychosocial need, and airway is the priority physical need.

C is incorrect because examining the throat may cause laryngospasm which can potentially be fatal. Further assessment is not needed at this time. The nurse must intervene to provide respiratory support.

Multiple Response

16. A 3-year-old girl has been diagnosed with strabismus. Which of the following signs does the nurse assess as manifestations of strabismus? (Select all that apply.)

    A. Closing one eye to see
    B. Excessive rubbing of eyes
    C. Tilting the head to one side to see
    D. Squinting to focus
    E. Sitting close to the TV
    F. Difficulty doing close-up work

    Rationale:

    Correct answers: A, C, D

    Strabismus (also known as "cross-eyed") is misalignment of the eyes due to either cranial nerve weakness, neuromuscular eye movement difficulty, or imbalance of extraocular muscles. The child with strabismus will close one eye, tilt the head to the side, or squint in order to focus.

    B is incorrect because excessive rubbing of the eyes is a manifestation of myopia (nearsightedness).

    E is incorrect because sitting close to the TV is a manifestation of myopia.

    F is incorrect because difficulty doing close-up work is a manifestation of hyperopia (farsightedness).

17. The nurse in the clinic is caring for a 9-year-old boy complaining of eye pain who was brought in by his parents. Which of the following symptoms would alert the nurse to a corneal abrasion? (Select all that apply.)

    A. Bloodshot eye

B. Increased tears
C. Unaffected vision
D. Ability to see well in bright light
E. Blurry vision

Rationale:

Correct answers: A, B, E

Corneal abrasions can occur with foreign bodies (dust, lint, sand) or when there is trauma to the cornea from a scratch or brushing against the eye. Symptoms of corneal abrasions include pain, stinging or burning, blurry vision, bloodshot eyes, swollen eyelids, increased tears, and foreign body sensation. Topical anesthetic or steroid eye drops can cause corneal abrasions as an adverse effect, so the eye should be patched when these drugs are being used. Corneal abrasion can also result from Bell's Palsy, so artificial tears should be used to keep the eye lubricated on the affected side.

C is incorrect because corneal abrasions usually affect vision temporarily and heal within a day or two.

D is incorrect because corneal abrasions often cause photosensitivity.

18. The parents of a 9-year-old girl diagnosed with amblyopia are learning about treatment options from the nurse. Which of the following treatments does the nurse inform the parents of? (Select all that apply.)

A. Glasses
B. Eye patch on the strong eye for 6 to 10 hours daily
C. Atropine drops in the weak eye
D. Surgery
E. Corticosteroid drops

Rationale:

Correct answers: A, D

Amblyopia (also known as "lazy eye") is misalignment of the eyes due to miscommunication between the eyes and the brain, most commonly caused by strabismus. The affected eye appears normal upon inspection, but vision is decreased. Treatment for strabismus includes glasses, eye patch over the strong eye, atropine drops in the strong eye, and corrective surgery.

B is incorrect because eye patching should only be used part-time, 4 to 6 hours daily to prevent reverse amblyopia from developing on the stronger eye.

C is incorrect because atropine drops are placed in the stronger eye as a treatment for amblyopia. (The atropine dilates the pupil of the stronger eye, making it difficult to see near, and forcing the weaker eye to strengthen.)

E is incorrect because corticosteroid drops are not commonly used to treat amblyopia. Ophthalmic corticosteroid medications are used to treat inflammation of the eye after ophthalmic surgery or other eye inflammation related to infections or damage to the eye from a chemical or foreign body.

19. The preoperative nurse is teaching the parents of a 3-year-old boy who is scheduled for bilateral myringotomy. Which of the following statements does the nurse include in the teaching? (Select all that apply.)

    A. "The procedure is performed under general anesthesia."
    B. "The surgeon will make a hole in the eardrum through which a small tube will be placed."
    C. "Your son will need to stay overnight after the procedure."

D. "You will need to bring your son back in 7 to 10 days to have the sutures removed."
E. "The tubes will likely stay in place for 6 to 18 months."

Rationale:

Correct answers: A, B, E

Bilateral myringotomy is an incision into the tympanic membrane, performed to relieve fluid collection from the middle ear, resulting in relief of pressure and drainage of purulent fluid. Small tubes are placed in holes created during surgery under general anesthesia, and the tubes fall out on their own after 6 to 18 months of being in place but must be surgically removed if the tubes remain in place longer than 2 years.

C is incorrect because this is generally an outpatient surgical procedure unless the child has significant medical history.

D is incorrect because no sutures are placed during a bilateral myringotomy.

20. The nurse in the family practice office is speaking with the parents of a 7-year-old girl diagnosed with frequent, recurring strep throat. Which of the following statements by the parents indicate the parents understand the tonsillectomy procedure?

A. "Our daughter will be given general anesthesia for the procedure."
B. "We will need to change her dressings the day after surgery."
C. "We will need to watch her for bleeding."
D. "She may not want to eat solid foods for about a week."
E. "We will bring her back in a week to have the stitches taken out."

Rationale:

Correct answers: A, C, D

Tonsillectomy is an outpatient procedure performed to remove the tonsils due to recurrent infection (tonsillitis), airway obstruction, or debris (tonsil stones). The procedure is performed under general anesthesia and takes approximately 20 minutes to perform. There is a risk for bleeding, which generally occurs the same day of surgery or in 7 to 10 days when the scabs come off. The throat is extremely sore for about a week after the surgery, and children usually do not eat solid foods during this time.

B is incorrect because the procedure is performed through the mouth and no dressing changes are required.

E is incorrect because no sutures are used in a tonsillectomy procedure.

21. The parents of a 9-month-old girl have brought her in to the clinic for acute otitis media. Which of the following manifestations does the nurse expect to find? (Select all that apply.)

    A. Pulling at the ear
    B. Irritability
    C. Hearty appetite
    D. Smiling and cooing
    E. Malaise
    F. Low temperature

Rationale:

Correct answers: A, B, E

Otitis media occurs when the eustachian tube is blocked due to nasal allergy attack or upper respiratory infection, causing fluid collection in the middle ear. Symptoms in infants and children include ear pain, pulling at the ear, irritability, rapid onset, malaise, and poor feeding.

C is incorrect because the nurse will expect the infant with otitis media to have a poor appetite, pain while bottle-feeding or breastfeeding, and decreased nutritional intake.

D is incorrect because the nurse will expect the infant with otitis media to be irritable.

F is incorrect because the nurse will expect to see an elevated temperature in an infant with otitis media.

22. A 7-year-old boy is in the clinic with his parents to see the nurse. The parents tell the nurse they believe he has trouble seeing. Which of the following signs indicate vision impairment in a child? (Select all that apply.)

    A. Imitation of facial expressions
    B. Frequent blinking
    C. Squinting
    D. Holding objects close
    E. Appropriate eye contact
    F. Tilting the head to the side to hear when someone whispers

Rationale:

Correct answers: B, C, D

Vision impairment can be due to several different factors, including amblyopia or strabismus, nearsightedness, sensory impairment, or corneal abrasion. Children with vision impairment will not be able to track objects, eye contact will be lacking, and they are unable to imitate facial expressions. The nurse will expect to observe the child squinting, holding objects close, and frequent blinking.

A is incorrect because the child with vision impairment is often unable to imitate facial expressions.

E is incorrect because the child with vision impairment is unable to make eye contact.

F is incorrect because this is a symptom of hearing loss, not impaired vision.

23. The nurse in the school clinic is caring for a 7-year-old girl who comes in for epistaxis. The nurse will initiate which of the following interventions? (Select all that apply.)

   A. Lie the child down on her back on the cot and have her apply pressure to the nostrils
   B. Apply heat to the bridge of the nose
   C. Keep the child calm
   D. Have the child sit upright with her head tilted forward
   E. Administer decongestant medication
   F. Perform nasal suctioning

Rationale:

Correct answers: C, D

Epistaxis is a nosebleed and can either be anterior or posterior, depending on where mucosa has been eroded and blood vessels are exposed. Interventions for epistaxis include keeping the child calm, having the child sit upright with their head tilted forward, and applying pressure to both nostrils below nasal bone. The parents should be notified that if interventions do not stop the bleeding, the healthcare provider should be contacted.

A is incorrect because when a child is experiencing epistaxis, lying the child down supine may allow blood to run down the nasopharynx and increase risk for aspiration.

B is incorrect because heat will cause vasodilation and increase blood flow to the area. An ice pack should be used instead.

E is incorrect because decongestant medication is not commonly used to treat epistaxis and may be unsafe for a 7-year-old child.

F is incorrect because epistaxis generally does not require nasal suctioning, and this is an inappropriate intervention for a school nurse to perform.

24. The nursing student in the pediatric clinic is learning about common causes of nasal obstruction in children. The nursing student learns about which of the following? (Select all that apply.)

    A. Foreign body
    B. Deviated septum
    C. Pharyngitis
    D. Rhinitis
    E. Epiglottitis
    F. Accumulation of nasal hairs

Rationale:

Correct answers: A, B, D

Nasal obstruction can be caused by rhinitis (inflammation of the mucosal lining of the nasal cavity), adenoid hypertrophy, foreign body, deviated septum, nasal polyps, hematoma, or tumors. Children with nasal obstruction are often mouth breathers, as the nasal cavity is blocked preventing breathing through the nose.

C is incorrect because pharyngitis is infection of the throat and does not cause nasal obstruction.

E is incorrect because epiglottitis is inflammation of the epiglottis and can be an airway emergency but does not cause nasal obstruction.

F is incorrect because children do not generally suffer from overgrowth or accumulation of nasal hairs.

25. A 4-year-old girl in the pediatric emergency room has been diagnosed with tonsillitis. When assessing the patient, which of the following symptoms does the nurse expect to find? (Select all that apply.)

A. Deep-red colored tonsils
B. Sore throat
C. Blood pressure 70/45
D. Swollen lymph nodes of the axillae
E. White or yellow film on tonsils

Rationale:

Correct answers: A, B, E

Tonsillitis is infection and inflammation of the tonsils. Symptoms include deep-red tonsils, sore throat, fever, swollen neck lymph nodes, and white or yellow film on the tonsils.

C is incorrect because this is hypotensive for a 4-year-old, and tonsillitis does not cause hypotension.

D is incorrect because lymph nodes of the neck are swollen in tonsillitis, not the axillae.

CHAPTER 2:

NCLEX-RN – PEDIATRIC: GROWTH AND DEVELOPMENT - 25 QUESTIONS

1. The nurse in the clinic is assessing communication patterns of a 5-month-old female patient. The nurse has determined the highest level of developing has been achieved if the child:

   A. Uses simple words like "dada"
   B. Uses monosyllabic babbling
   C. Links syllables together
   D. Coos when comforted

   Rationale:
   Correct answer: B

   Monosyllabic babbling is expected to occur between the ages of 3 and 6 months.

   A is incorrect because simple words like "dada" is expected to occur between the ages of 9 and 12 months.

   C is incorrect because linking of syllables is expected to occur between the ages of 6 and 9 months.

D is incorrect because cooing starts at birth and continues until approximately 2 months.

2. The nurse in the clinic is speaking with the mother of an 8-year-old girl who is 4 feet tall. The nurse tells the mother the best car safety device for her daughter is which of the following?

   A. Front-facing convertible seat with a harness
   B. Rear-facing convertible seat
   C. Regular seat in the car with the seat belt firmly across the body, from one shoulder down to the opposite hip
   D. Booster seat with belt-positioning belt

Rationale:

Correct answer: D

The American Academy of Pediatrics (AAP) recommends a booster seat with a belt-positioning belt is to be used for children between the ages of 8 and 12 years old and until they have reached at least 4 feet, 9 inches tall. The belt should lie across the middle of the chest, not near the neck or face.

A is incorrect because a front-facing convertible seats with a harness is used until age 5 or when the upper weight or height limit of the convertible seat has been reached.

B is incorrect because the AAP recommends that toddlers are kept in rear-facing car seats until age 2, or until they reach the maximum height and weight for their seat.

C is incorrect because the regular seat belt should not be used until the child is 4 feet, 9 inches tall.

3. The student nurse is learning about pediatric growth and development. The student nurse learns which developmental stage is unstable and challenging regarding personal identity development?

   A. Adolescence
   B. Toddlerhood
   C. School-age
   D. Infancy

Rationale:

Correct answer: A

Adolescence (age 12 to 20) is an unstable, challenging time for developing personal identity as many things are occurring, including life choices, physical changes, cognitive changes, and social changes. Erikson coined this identity crisis as “identity versus role confusion” as it is a turning point in the life of the individual and is a critical part of development. The positive outcome for this stage is developing a coherent sense of self with plans for future work or education. If the adolescent demonstrates an inability to develop a personal and vocational identity, this is the negative outcome for this stage.

B is incorrect because toddlers (age 1 to 3) have not developed personal identity yet. The developmental task at this stage is “autonomy vs. shame and doubt.” The positive outcome for the child is exercising self-control and having the ability to control her environment directly.

C is incorrect because the school-age child (age 6 to 12) is characterized by simple, observable personal identity (boy, girl, child, good, etc.). The developmental task is “industry versus inferiority.” The positive outcome is developing a sense of confidence and using creativity to influence the environment.

D is incorrect because infancy is characterized by identifying faces of mother, father, etc. The task is "trust versus mistrust."

4. A 15-year-old boy has been admitted to the hospital for acute appendicitis and is recovering from appendectomy. Which nursing intervention is most appropriate regarding facilitation of normal growth and development?

   A. Allow the family to bring the boy his favorite computer games
   B. Encourage the parents to sleep in the room with the boy
   C. Encourage the boy to read, rest, and make his own food choices
   D. Allow the boy to participate in group activities with other same-age individuals when medically stable

Rationale:

Correct answer: D

Adolescents seek autonomy and independence and are sometimes unsure about spending time with their parents when hospitalized. Peer group is important, and separation from their friends can cause anxiety. Allowing the child time to spend with others of a similar age can be beneficial for facilitating normal development.

A is incorrect because, although electronics may be enjoyable to the boy, this may isolate the teen from his peer group. Promoting social interaction is a greater priority than encouraging use of favorite toys and games.

B is incorrect because having the parents sleep in the room does not promote interaction with peers and may not be the boy's desire. The nurse should talk with the boy first to determine if he wants his parents to stay in the room, and then talk with the parents to help develop a plan that both the boy and the parents are comfortable with.

C is incorrect because encouraging rest and solitary activities, such as reading, may isolate the teen from their peer group. Allowing the boy to make his own food choices may not meet dietary needs for normal growth.

5. The nurse in the clinic is evaluating a 24-month boy's developmental level. Which observation does the nurse expect?

   A. Copies a circle
   B. Uses a cup when drinking
   C. Skips and hops on one foot
   D. Walks alone, throws objects, has a 10-word vocabulary

   Rationale:

   Correct answer: B

   By the age of 24 months, a child should be able to use a spoon and drink from a cup, although some spilling may occur. Other milestones common for a 24-month-old include building a 5 to 6 block tower, having a 300-word vocabulary, and obeying easy commands.

   A is incorrect because the ability to copy a circle occurs at age 3 years.

   C is incorrect because a child is not expected to skip and hop on one foot until the age of 4 years.

   D is incorrect because these are expectations for a child between the ages of 15 and 18 months.

6. The nurse in the clinic is interviewing a mother who expresses concern regarding her 3-year-old daughter demanding a bottle of milk in her bed at naptime and bedtime. What is the most appropriate suggestion the nurse should give?

A. "Try giving your daughter milk in a sippy-cup before the nap, instead of a bottle in the bed."
B. "Give your daughter the bottle of milk at naptime but not bedtime."
C. "You can give your daughter the bottle if it contains 50 percent juice and 50 percent water inside."
D. "You can give your daughter the bottle if it has water in it."

Rationale:

Correct answer: A

The American Academy of Pediatrics (AAP) recommends weaning a baby from the bottle by 18 months of age. Toddlers should not be given bottles or cups to fall asleep with if they contain milk, juice, or any other sweetened beverage, as it increases risk of dental caries. The best way to help wean this child from the bottle at age 3 is to offer the desired beverage in a sippy-cup, before laying her down.

B is incorrect because the AAP recommends weaning the bedtime bottle last, because it's usually the hardest for the child to give up.

C is incorrect because watered-down juice can cause dental caries.

D is incorrect because, although water is safer for the teeth than milk or juice, a 3-year-old should transition to the sippy-cup instead of the bottle.

7. A 5-year-old boy with a fractured femur is on the pediatric orthopedic unit in traction. When planning the boy's care, which of the following activities does the nurse include?

   A. Large picture books
   B. A radio
   C. Crayons and coloring book
   D. Sports videos

Rationale:

Correct answer: C

The preschooler engages in simple and imaginative play including coloring books and crayons, felt and magnetic boards, puppets, and Play-Doh. While in traction, the nurse should encourage activities that hold the child's interest and encourage imagination and creativity. The child must be reminded not to turn to either side while in traction, so the coloring supplies should be placed within easy reach on the over-bed table.

A is incorrect because infants and toddlers enjoy large picture books.

B is incorrect because a 5-year-old may not know how to operate a radio. This is more appropriate for an adolescent.

D is incorrect because sports videos are appropriate for an adolescent, not a school-age child.

8. The nurse in the clinic works with children of all ages regularly. Which of the following age groups does the nurse know has a tendency to have eating disorders?

    A. Adolescents
    B. Toddlers
    C. School-age children
    D. Infants

Rationale:

Correct answer: A

Eating disorders include anorexia nervosa, bulimia, and binge eating. Adolescents (age 12-20) are undergoing many changes, including mental, physical, cognitive, and social. They are highly impressionable and easily affected by the thoughts and feelings of others, while exerting their independence from parents. Body image becomes more important during adolescence than previously in life. Pressure may be felt by the adolescent with all the changes around them, and eating disorders are an attempt at gaining control.

B is incorrect because toddlers (age 1 to 3) do not exhibit eating disorders.

C is incorrect because school-age children (6 to 12) rarely exhibit eating disorders. Older school-age girls do tend to develop body image concerns, but eating disorders are more common after the age of 12 than before.

D is incorrect because infants (birth to 12 months) do not exhibit eating disorders.

9. The mother of a 3-year-old girl tells the nurse in the family practice clinic that her daughter is rebellious and throws temper tantrums. Which response by the nurse is most appropriate?

   A. "Punish the child for saying "no" in order to change her behavior."
   B. "In order to reduce your stress, you should allow this behavior because it is normal for this age. She will grow out of it."
   C. "We can talk about how to set limits on your daughter's behavior."
   D. "Ignore your daughter completely when she acts in this manner. When she sees that she is not gaining your attention, she will stop."

Rationale:

Correct answer: C

Children's focus is on independence from ages 1 to 3 years, according to Erikson. This often means rebelling against parent wishes and saying "no" as well as throwing temper tantrums. The parents must be consistent in setting limits that allow the child to have some independence and control over their environment, while learning self-control.

A is incorrect because saying "no" is normal behavior at this age. It is more appropriate for the nurse to teach the mother how to set limits in order to effectively control her child's behavior.

B is incorrect because although this behavior *is* normal, this statement is dismissive and does not teach the parent how to deal with the behavior or to set limits.

D is incorrect because ignoring the child during rebellious activity or temper tantrums is not safe for the child.

10. The nurse in the clinic works with patients of all ages. The nurse knows the age group that demonstrates regression when experiencing sickness is which of the following?

    A. Adolescent
    B. Young adult
    C. Toddler
    D. Infant

Rationale:

Correct answer: C

Regression is backtracking to a previous milestone or earlier level of functioning. Toddlers are beginning to demonstrate independence from parents, and when ill, the toddler may be unable to do certain things on their own. Regression is seen as the toddler tending to depend more on the parents and perform at earlier developmental levels (toilet training, sleeping, etc.) until the illness is resolved.

A is incorrect because adolescents do not typically demonstrate regression with illness.

B is incorrect because young adults do not typically demonstrate regression with illness.

D is incorrect because infants do not typically demonstrate regression with illness.

11. A 2-year-old was admitted for illness 6 days ago, and the parents visited the child briefly every evening. For the first 2 days, the child cried and was inconsolable. During the next 3 days, the child became quiet and withdrawn. Today, the child is in the hospital playroom when her parents come to visit. The child does not run to her parents when they arrive but continues to play with building blocks with the hospital volunteer. How does the nurse interpret this behavior?

    A. The child is still withdrawn
    B. The child is self-centered
    C. The child is experiencing despair
    D. The child is behaving as expected

Rationale:

Correct answer: D

Young children progress through several stages of separation anxiety when separated from their parents. These phases are protest, despair, and denial/detachment. This child is behaving normally for the detachment phase, showing interest in the environment and hospital staff. These stages occur as a result of lack of physical connection between the child and the parents.

A is incorrect because the child is playing, which is not a sign of withdrawal. A child who acts withdrawn is in the despair stage of separation anxiety.

B is incorrect because self-centeredness is not a stage of separation anxiety.

C is incorrect because the child was in despair during days 3 to 5 of the hospital stay. A child in the despair stage of separation anxiety appears subdued, apathetic, picks at food, and is uninterested in the surrounding environment.

12. A 16-year-old boy is admitted for an illness. According to Erikson, which intervention does the nurse implement?

    A. Encourage the boy to invite his friends to visit
    B. Encourage the parents to help the boy keep up with material being covered at school
    C. Offer the boy a visit from pastoral care
    D. Discourage the use of electronics

Rationale:

Correct answer: A

Erikson developed the theory of psychosocial development consisting of eight stages beginning at infancy and progressing to adulthood. Erikson's theory states that during adolescence (age 12 to 20) the developmental task is "identity versus role confusion." The most important people in this age group are the boy's peers. Encouraging the friends to visit will help keep the boy from becoming withdrawn and socially isolated.

B is incorrect because physical and social interaction with peers is more important than schoolwork for the ill adolescent. If his needs for interaction with his peer group are met, he will be more likely to keep up with his schoolwork.

C is incorrect because social groups are generally more important to adolescents than spiritual matters.

D is incorrect because, although electronic devices can cause isolation, they can also be a source of connecting with the peer group through social media. Per hospital policy and with the parents' permission, the nurse should allow the boy to use electronics and also encourage social interaction with visitors.

13. The nurse on the maternity unit is providing discharge instructions to the mother of an infant regarding physical and psychosocial development. Which of the following instructions is appropriate for the nurse to give?

    A. Allow the infant to signal needs
    B. The baby's birth weight should be doubled by 12 months of age
    C. Allow the infant to cry for 3 to 5 minutes before intervening
    D. Expect teething to begin around 3 to 4 months

Rationale:

Correct answer: A

Erikson developed the theory of psychosocial development consisting of eight stages beginning at infancy and progressing to adulthood. Erikson's theory of psychosocial development states the newborn must be allowed to signal needs in order to learn how to control the environment. Some common infant signals include rubbing the eyes while tired, turning the head away when the baby needs a break from eye contact, and crying when tired or when needing to have a bowel movement.

B is incorrect because an infant's birth weight should double by 5 months old and triple by 12 months of age.

C is incorrect because the developmental task in infancy (birth to 12 months) is trust versus mistrust. Delayed response by the caregiver when the infant cries leads to mistrust.

D is incorrect because, although some babies start teething earlier, the mother should not expect the beginning of teething until about 6 months of age.

14. The nurse is teaching a childcare and parenting class to expecting parents. When one of the expectant parents asks the nurse about Sudden Infant Death Syndrome (SIDS), what the most appropriate response by the nurse?
    A. "Using a pacifier while sleeping increases the risk for SIDS."
    B. "Child abuse in the form of intentional suffocation is often misdiagnosed as SIDS and may make up nearly 50 percent of reported SIDS cases."
    C. "Overheating and exposure to tobacco smoke are known to increase the risk for SIDS, which is the leading cause of death between 1 and 12 months."
    D. "The most effective way to prevent SIDS is to put all babies to sleep on their backs when under the age of 6 months."

Rationale:

Correct answer: C

SIDS is the most common cause of death in infancy, while the cause is not always known. Expecting mothers should be taught not to smoke or be exposed to tobacco smoke during pregnancy. Parents of infants must be taught to place the child on the back to sleep, not to use heavy blankets or covers and not to place the infant in the bed with them in order to decrease the risk of SIDS.

A is incorrect because use of a pacifier decreases the risk for SIDS.

B is incorrect because these misdiagnosed child abuse cases only make up about 5 percent of SIDS cases.

D is incorrect because babies should be laid on their back to sleep for the first 12 months of life to prevent SIDS.

15. The nurse on the pediatric unit is observing children in the playroom. The nurse would expect to see 5-year-old children playing in which of the following manners?

    A. Board games with school-age children
    B. With their toys alongside other children, without interacting much
    C. Playing with push-pull toys and stuffed animals
    D. Cooperatively with other preschoolers

Rationale:

Correct answer: D

Preschoolers (age 3 to 6 years) typically play cooperatively with others of the same age group. Interactive play generally starts around the age of 5 years. Preschoolers typically enjoy playground toys, tricycles (with helmet), coloring activities, matching games, and housekeeping toys that allow them to imitate adult professions and activities.

A is incorrect because competitive play is typical seen with older children, not preschoolers.

B is incorrect because this describes parallel play, which is typical of toddlers (age 1 to 3 years).

C is incorrect because this describes play characteristic of toddlers (age 1 to 3 years).

16. The nurse is providing education to the parents of a 13-year-old boy. Which of the following statements is the most important for the nurse to make?

A. “Motor vehicle accidents are the most common cause of death among adolescents, so teach him to wear his seatbelt while driving.”
B. “The sexual education that children receive in school may not be sufficient. Discussions should continue at home regarding sexual abstinence, safe sex, and sexually transmitted infections (STIs).”
C. “It is important to be aware of the signs of marijuana use because use has increased among middle-schoolers in the last five years.”
D. “It is important to have your child screened by a cardiologist because heart disease is on the rise amongst teenagers.”

Rationale:

Correct answer: B

Children often begin to learn about sex in school in the fifth grade. Discussions should continue throughout adolescence to help children develop their knowledge about the anatomy and physiology of the human body as well as the potential consequences of teenage sexual experiences (peer pressure, unwanted pregnancies, difficult relationships, STIs.) The pediatric nurse should make themselves available to discuss these issues with the parents and/or the child.

A is incorrect because although accidents (unintentional injuries) are the leading cause of death among adolescents, this child is only 13 years old and will not be driving for several years. (Note: motor vehicle accidents account for one-third of all deaths to teenagers.)

C is incorrect because marijuana use among middle-school children has actually decreased recently, despite changes in laws.

D is incorrect because unless specific symptoms are assessed, a 13-year-old boy does not need to be screened by a cardiologist.

17. The nurse on the pediatric unit is caring for an adolescent admitted for pneumonia. The nurse knows the major threat experienced by the adolescent who is hospitalized is which of the following?

    A. Pain management
    B. Restricted physical activity
    C. Altered body image
    D. Separation from family

Rationale:

Correct answer: C

Body image is very important to the adolescent. Hospitalization, especially if it requires IVs and specialized equipment, or weight loss from prolonged illness, can be traumatic to the individual.

A is incorrect because pain management is important to the adolescent but not as concerning as body image.

B is incorrect because restricted physical activity affects the adolescent, but body image and their peer group are often the greater concerns.

D is incorrect because separation from family affects the adolescent but is not the major threat. Adolescents are often even more tied to their peer group than they are to their family.

18. The pediatric nurse is caring for a 5-month-old infant in the family practice clinic. At birth, the baby weighed 6 lbs. 11 oz. What does the nurse expect the baby's weight to be now?

    A. It depends on whether the baby is breastfed or formula-fed.
    B. 15 lbs. 8 oz.
    C. 20 lbs. 1 oz.
    D. 13 lbs. 6 oz.

Rationale:

Correct answer: D

An infant's birth weight should double by the age of 5 months.

A is incorrect because regardless of whether the baby is fed formula or breastmilk, the weight should double by 5 months of age.

B is incorrect because 15 lbs. 8 oz. is more than double the birthweight, which is not expected at this time.

C is incorrect because 20 lbs. 1 oz. represents triple the birth weight, which should be reached by 12 months of age.

19. A nurse is working with children and adolescents on the pediatric ward of the hospital. The nurse knows the individual's development of distinguishing right and wrong and developing ethical values on which to base actions is which of the following?

    A. Moral development
    B. Cognitive development
    C. Psychosocial development
    D. Psychoanalytic development

Rationale:

Correct answer: A

Moral development is learning to distinguish right and wrong as well as acquiring ethical values to base actions on.

B is incorrect because cognitive development is knowledge and learning.

C is incorrect because psychosocial development is learning one's role in society.

D is incorrect because psychoanalytic development is development of personality.

20. The nurse is developing a care plan for an adolescent girl admitted for pneumonia. Which statement regarding normal growth and development is effective nursing care is based on?

    A. Growth occurs at same rates for individuals in the same stage
    B. Development progresses from complex to simple tasks
    C. Individuals have unique growth patterns and development that are difficult to predict
    D. Success in each phase of growth and development affects ability to successfully complete subsequent phases

Rationale:

Correct answer: D

Developmental failures can result in deficiencies in later developmental stages. The nurse must be alert to developmental stages in order to understand patient growth and development.

A is incorrect because growth patterns vary between individuals in the same stage.

B is incorrect because development progresses from simple to complex tasks.

C is incorrect because growth and development patterns vary from one individual to another but are predictable within a normal range for age and gender.

21. The nurse in the clinic is caring for school-age children. The nurse knows physical growth involves which of the following?

    A. Skill level changes
    B. Skeletal structure strengthening
    C. Improved intellectual task performance
    D. Learning appropriate responses to social situations

Rationale:

Correct answer: B

Physical growth includes height, weight, bones, and teeth changes and is objective and measurable.

A is incorrect because skill level changes describe physical and intellectual development, not growth.

C is incorrect because improved intellectual task performance describes cognitive development.

D is incorrect because responses to social situations describes psychosocial development.

22. The nursing student on the pediatric ward is learning about development. Which of the following does the student identify as development?

   A. 7-month-old pulls up to standing position
   B. 8-month-old develops two lower teeth
   C. Infant birth weight doubles by 6 months
   D. Young child uses words to make needs known instead of crying

Rationale:

Correct answer: A

An infant pulling up to standing position demonstrates change in function and skill, which is development and occurs predictably (i.e., infant sits up, pulls up, then stands).

B is incorrect because development of teeth is demonstrative of growth.

C is incorrect because doubling of infant birth weight is demonstrative of growth.

D is incorrect because developing communication skills to express needs demonstrates maturation.

23. A mother and father are in the clinic speaking with the nurse about their 2-year-old son. The child is very independent and rejects authority of the parents. The nurse should respond based on which of the following?

A. The parents must tighten control on their child
B. The need for autonomy is usually apparent by puberty
C. Punishment and limiting the child's choices will restore trust
D. Independence demonstrated by their child is normal and part of maturation

Rationale:

Correct answer: D

Children in this developmental stage learn self-care and develop autonomy. The toddler years mark the beginning of establishing independence. Parents should be encouraged to set limits and allow the child to make simple choices to gain a feeling of control over their environment. ("What shirt would you like to wear today? Do you want bananas or peas with your lunch?")

A is incorrect because children at this stage need supervision and opportunities to make choices for themselves, not strict control.

B is incorrect because the need for autonomy appears between ages 1 and 3 years, long before puberty.

C is incorrect because punishment and limiting the child's choices can create shame and doubt in the child.

24. The nurse on the pediatric medical-surgical unit is caring for an adolescent admitted for fractures. The nurse knows this adolescent's developmental needs are best met by which of the following interventions?

A. Providing word puzzles and other diversional activities

B. Providing privacy when the adolescent's significant other comes to visit
C. Encouraging parents to stay with the adolescent all the time
D. Explaining procedures and including the adolescent in the decision-making process

Rationale:

Correct answer: D

Meeting an adolescent's developmental needs includes allowing participation in decisions regarding care. Adolescents need to understand issues regarding their treatment and tend to cooperate and cope better if they are involved in the decision-making process.

A is incorrect because diversional activities are appropriate for school-aged children.

B is incorrect because privacy during the significant other's visits is appropriate for the young adult.

C is incorrect because adolescents need parental presence as well as independence and separation. It is important for the nurse to talk with both the patient and the parents to determine how much time of parental visitation is desired and to help balance the child's desires with the parent's wishes.

25. The nursing student in the family clinic is learning about Piaget's theory of cognitive development. The student learns that the school age child, age 7 to 11 years, demonstrates concrete operations when which of the following is demonstrated?

    A. Begins to think abstractly
    B. Participates in parallel play
    C. Can communicate with others at a simple level

D. Recognizes others perceive things differently

Rationale:

Correct answer: D

Piaget developed the theory of cognitive development, which describes the child's mental model of how they see the world. Age 7 to 11 years, or concrete operations stage, according to Piaget, is characterized by the ability to think through processes without performing them and mentally understanding others' viewpoints if different from their own.

A is incorrect because abstract thought is apparent in an older child, age 11 years on.

B is incorrect because parallel play is demonstrated by younger children, 2 to 5 years.

C is incorrect because simple level communication is demonstrated up to age 7 years.

CHAPTER 3:

NCLEX-RN – PEDIATRIC: NEUROLOGY - 25 QUESTIONS

1. The nurse in the pediatric intensive care unit (ICU) is caring for an infant with a congenital myelomeningocele. The nurse knows this condition is commonly associated with which of the following?

    A. Hydrocephalus
    B. Microencephaly
    C. Cranial suture overlap
    D. Absence of cranial vault

Rationale:

Correct answer: A

Congenital myelomeningocele is a defect of the neural tube that develops in utero and causes the fetal spinal bones to incompletely form and thus fail to completely cover the spinal cord. The spinal cord and meninges protrude from the child's back. The condition is commonly associated with hydrocephalus, or excessive cerebrospinal fluid (CSF) in the cranial vault.

B is incorrect because microencephaly is associated with maternal exposure to rubella or cytomegalovirus (CMV).

C is incorrect because cranial suture overlap may occur with a vaginal birth but is not associated with myelomeningocele.

D is incorrect because absence of cranial vault or anencephaly is an unrelated neural tube defect.

2. An infant is brought to the emergency room for unusual behavior. The pediatric nurse assesses for which of the following manifestations that could indicate increased intracranial pressure?

   A. Overflow voiding
   B. Bulging fontanel with crying
   C. High-pitched cry
   D. Minimal movement of lower extremities

Rationale:

Correct answer: C

Intracranial pressure is the pressure within the skull. Increased intracranial pressure can cause brain injury or be the result of brain injury (most commonly caused by shaken baby syndrome). Increased intracranial pressure in an infant is usually indicated by a high-pitched cry, most notably with Chiari malformation obstructing CSF flow. Nausea, vomiting, decreased level of consciousness, and sluggish or non-reactive pupils are other signs of increased ICP.

A is incorrect because overflow voiding is associated with neurogenic bladder.

B is incorrect because a bulging fontanel when the infant cries is a normal finding and not indicating of increased ICP.

D is incorrect because minimal movement of lower extremities is associated with damage to the spinal cord.

3. The nurse in the neonatal intensive care unit (NICU) is caring for a newborn with open spinal defect. When the parents arrive to meet their infant for the first time, which of the following is a priority nursing action?

   A. Encourage the parents to feed the newborn
   B. Discuss parental fears and concerns
   C. Provide educational pamphlets
   D. Emphasize normal and positive features of the newborn

Rationale

Correct answer: D

An open spinal defect is a defect of the neural tube that develops in utero and causes the fetus' spinal bones to form incompletely. The spinal bones and meninges fail to completely cover the spinal cord, which requires surgical intervention. Parents of children with disability or defect need to hear positive comments and emphasis on the normal and beautiful aspects of their child. The nurse must teach the parents how to hold the child, if possible, and encourage bonding and positive interaction.

A is incorrect because feeding of the infant must wait until after the defect is repaired.

B is incorrect because discussion of fears and concerns is not priority during the first visit.

C is incorrect because educational material is not priority for the first visit.

4. The nurse in the clinic is speaking with the parents of a newborn male with Down syndrome. Which of the following would be the most appropriate statement for the nurse to make when teaching the parents about the baby's diagnosis?

A. “Plan to teach the child something new daily as he grows up, so he can be as independent as possible.”
B. “The life expectancy for children with Down syndrome is significantly longer than it used to be.”
C. “Large ears and long fingers are common with Down syndrome.”
D. “If your child doesn’t learn to read by the age of 6, he will probably never read.”

Rationale:

Correct answer: B

Down syndrome is a genetic defect that occurs when an extra chromosome is inherited. Down syndrome causes decreased muscle tone, large forehead, flattened facial features, congenital heart defects, and intellectual disability. When Down syndrome was first discovered, children often did not live beyond age 15. In the 1980s, the life expectancy was 25 years. The current life expectancy is age 60.

No cure is available for Down’s syndrome, but many treatments are available to enhance quality of life and promote healthy, active and more independent lives. Many people with Down syndrome can still learn the physical, mental, and social skills that most other people acquire; they just do it at a different pace.

A is incorrect because learning new things daily may not be possible for a child with Down syndrome.

C is incorrect because small ears and short fingers are characteristic with Down syndrome.

D is incorrect because all children with Down’s syndrome will have some degree of learning disability. The ability to communicate or to read may develop later than other children the same age. It is important for the nurse to provide factual information to prepare the parents for life with a child with Down syndrome.

5. The nurse is walking a 6-year-old child with a seizure disorder back from the restroom in his hospital room. When the child starts exhibiting tonic-clonic movements, what is the first action the nurse should take?

   A. Note the time
   B. Ease the child to the floor
   C. Clear the area of objects and pad the child's head
   D. Roll child to the side-lying position for airway protection

Rationale:

Correct answer: A

A tonic-clonic seizure is characterized by stiffened muscles, jerking movements, and loss of consciousness. The time should be noted quickly for the nurse to be able to calculate how long the seizure lasts. After noting the time, the nurse's greatest priority is to stay with the patient and provide for safety, while monitoring the airway.

B is incorrect because easing the child to the floor is the first action after noting the start time.

C is incorrect because clearing the area and padding the child's head is important but not the first action. Risk for injury is increased during a tonic-clonic seizure, and safety is the greatest priority after noting the start time of the seizure.

D is incorrect because rolling the child to a side-lying position to protect the airway is important during a tonic-clonic seizure but should not be done until after the start time is noted, the patient has been eased to the floor, and the head has been padded.

6. The nurse in the pediatric emergency room is assessing a child who sustained a moderate brain injury after a fall. Which assessment gives

the earliest indication of potential increasing intracranial pressure (ICP) in this child?

A. Bilateral pupil response to light
B. Vital signs
C. Level of consciousness
D. Gross motor strength

Rationale:

Correct answer: C

Brain injury is caused by several actions including violent shaking, a direct blow, whiplash, or a fall and results in shaking of the brain and trauma. Changes in level of consciousness are the earliest indicator of increasing ICP in a child because brain cells responsible for cognition are extremely sensitive to decreased circulating oxygen in cerebral blood flow.

A is incorrect because changes in level of consciousness (disorientation, restlessness) are the earliest indicator of increasing ICP and may be seen before changes in pupillary response are assessed.

B is incorrect because changes in vital signs are a later sign of increasing ICP. Vital sign changes that correlate with increasing ICP include decreased pulse and respiratory rate, increase in blood pressure and temperature, widened pulse pressure, and Cheyne-stokes breathing (rhythmic waxing and waning of rate and depth of respirations alternating with brief periods of apnea).

D is incorrect because gross motor strength (weakness on one extremity or on one side of the body) usually occurs after changes in level of consciousness.

7. A child in the pediatric neurological intensive care unit (NICU) has mannitol prescribed by the healthcare provider for head injury. Which of the following best indicates the medication is effective?

   A. Increased urine output
   B. Improved level of consciousness (LOC)
   C. Decreased facial swelling
   D. Intracranial pressure (ICP) 22 mm Hg

Rationale:

Correct answer: B

Increased ICP is manifested by altered level of consciousness (LOC), headache, nausea and vomiting, pupillary changes, diplopia, increased systolic blood pressure, slow respirations, slow and bounding pulse, widening pulse pressure, and hyper/hypothermia. Mannitol is an osmotic diuretic that decreases intracranial pressure. LOC would be the best indicator of the medication being an effective treatment.

A is incorrect because increased urine output is expected with an osmotic diuretic, but the effectiveness is best assessed by improved LOC.

C is incorrect because although an osmotic diuretic may decrease facial swelling, the medication is not primarily given for the purpose of reducing edema.

D is incorrect because normal ICP is 10-20 mm Hg. Increased ICP is not a sign that mannitol is effective, as this is a high reading.

8. The nurse on the pediatric intensive care unit (ICU) is admitting a 10-year-old girl for a suspected infratentorial brain tumor. Which action is the nurse's greatest priority?

   A. Implement seizure precautions
   B. Introduce the child to other patients of the same age

C. Prepare the child and her parents for the ordered diagnostic procedures
D. Use distraction techniques to eliminate the child's anxiety

Rationale:

Correct answer: C

Infratentorial brain tumors, including glial tumors and medulloblastomas, are located in the cerebellum or brain stem and affect movement coordination, problem solving, judgement, personality, and reasoning. The diagnosis of suspected an infratentorial brain tumor requires diagnostic procedures to confirm, so the nurse should prepare the family.

It is the ordering healthcare provider's responsibility to explain the diagnostic procedure and obtain consent, but the nurse must be available to answer questions and perform the pre-procedure preparations for the client. These preparations may include switching the child to a gown without snaps (if going for an MRI), administering pre-procedure medications, initiating IV access, performing a neurological assessment, documenting vital signs, and reinforcing the teaching provided by the ordering healthcare provider.

A is incorrect because infratentorial brain tumors do not commonly cause seizure activity.

B is incorrect because promoting social interaction with other children of the same age meets the child's psychosocial needs. The greater nursing priority is to prepare the child and family for diagnostic procedures, which are a greater physical need at this time.

D is incorrect because anxiety may be reduced with distraction, but diagnostic procedures are the greatest priority.

9. The nurse in the clinic is assessing an 8-year-old boy who complains of a sore throat, generally not feeling well, muscle tenderness, bilateral leg weakness, and recent tingling in the fingertips. Which assessment is most important for the nurse to assess?

   A. 24-hour previous dietary intake
   B. Exposure to contagious illnesses
   C. Urination difficulty
   D. Swallowing ability

Rationale:

Correct answer: D

The child has symptoms of Guillain-Barre (GB) syndrome, a progressive inflammatory autoimmune response occurring in the peripheral nervous system, in which paralysis ascends from the lower extremities upward. With GB syndrome, nerve roots are compressed, and demyelination occurs. A sore throat commonly precedes paralysis related to this condition. Swallowing ability should be evaluated to determine if immediate action is needed.

A is incorrect because 24-hour dietary intake will not elicit useful information related to the symptoms. Assessment of the airway (right-here-and-now) is a greater priority than previous food intake.

B is incorrect because the child is showing signs of GB, which is not contagious.

C is incorrect because difficulty with urination will not elicit useful information related to the symptoms, and the urinary system does not take priority over the airway.

10. A 13-year-old male patient in the pediatric intensive care unit (ICU) was admitted the previous day following a motor vehicle accident. When

assessing the adolescent, which finding indicates spinal shock is resolving?

A. Widening pulse pressure
B. Hyperactive reflexes
C. Atonic urinary bladder
D. Flaccid paralysis

Rationale:

Correct answer: B

Spinal shock is manifested by bradycardia, decreased pulses, hypotension, complete loss of sensation, and vasodilation with warm skin. After spinal cord injury and spinal shock, nerve reflex return usually results in hyperactivity and spasticity of limbs and bladder. Abnormally strong reflexes can be produced with minimal stimulation.

A is incorrect because widened pulse pressure is unrelated to resolution of spinal shock and may be an indication of increasing intracranial pressure.

C is incorrect because atonic urinary bladder is an indication of continuing spinal shock.

D is incorrect because flaccid paralysis of skeletal muscles is an effect of spinal shock, indicating it is not yet resolving.

11. The nurse in the pediatric emergency room is caring for a 9-year-old girl with suspected Guillain-Barre (GB) syndrome. Which of the following is not a symptom associated with this syndrome?

    A. Weakening or tingling sensation in legs
    B. Weakness in arms and upper body
    C. Nearly complete paralysis
    D. Altered mental status

Rationale:

Correct answer: D

Guillain-Barre syndrome is a progressive inflammatory autoimmune disorder occurring in the peripheral nervous system, in which paralysis ascends from the lower extremities upward. With GB syndrome, nerve roots are compressed, and demyelination occurs. Complete paralysis can occur over time. Physical movement and sensation are affected, but altered mental status is not a symptom associated with Guillain-Barre.

A is incorrect because weakening or tingling sensation in the legs is a symptom of Guillain-Barre.

B is incorrect because weakness in arms and upper body is a symptom of Guillain-Barre.

C is incorrect because nearly complete paralysis is a symptom of Guillain-Barre.

12. The nurse in the family practice clinic is teaching the parents of a 4-year-old about epilepsy. Which of the following is NOT a test that can diagnose epilepsy?

    A. Positron Emission Tomography (PET) scan
    B. Electroencephalogram (EEG)
    C. Magnetic resonance imaging (MRI) of the brain
    D. Wada test

Rationale:

Correct answer: D

Epilepsy is a disorder of the neurological system characterized by loss of consciousness, convulsions, and recurrent episodes of disturbance of sensory functions due to abnormal brain electrical activity. A Wada test itself does not diagnose epilepsy. After epilepsy is diagnosed, a Wada test can be used to determine which hemisphere controls language and helps the neurosurgeon plan the surgical intervention for epilepsy.

A is incorrect because a PET scan can diagnose epilepsy.

B is incorrect because an electroencephalogram (EEG) charts and records the electrical activity in the brain. Certain abnormal patterns, such as spike and sharp wave activities on an EEG, can help support or confirm a clinical diagnosis of epilepsy.

C is incorrect because MRI of the brain can be used to diagnose epilepsy.

13. The family of a 6-year-old girl diagnosed with epilepsy asks the nurse how epilepsy can be treated to eliminate or reduce seizure frequency. Which of the following does the nurse NOT inform the parents of?

    A. Cognitive-behavioral therapy
    B. Narrow spectrum and broad-spectrum antiepileptic medications
    C. Vagus nerve stimulation
    D. Surgery

Rationale:

Correct answer: A

Epilepsy is a disorder of the neurological system characterized by loss of consciousness, convulsions, and recurrent episodes of disturbance of sensory functions due to abnormal brain electrical activity. Behavioral or emotional difficulty may develop in response to stigmatization, so cognitive-behavioral therapy is not usually considered to eliminate or reduce seizure frequency; however. it may be used as adjunctive therapy.

B is incorrect because narrow- and broad-spectrum antiepileptic medications are used for treatment of epilepsy.

C is incorrect because vagus nerve stimulation is used for treatment of epilepsy.

D is incorrect because surgery is used for treatment of epilepsy.

14. The nurse in the pediatric intensive care unit (PICU) is caring for an infant diagnosed with hydrocephalus. When teaching the parents about treatments for hydrocephalus, which of the following does the nurse inform the parents of as a possibility?

    A. Lumbar puncture
    B. Osmotic diuretics
    C. Shunt placement
    D. Monitoring intracranial pressure

Rationale:

Correct answer: C

Hydrocephalus is accumulation of the spinal fluid within the brain due to abnormal production or recycling of the fluid in the neurological system. This leads to rapid enlargement of the head and neurological disruption. A shunt can be placed in the brain or the abdomen to create a cerebrospinal fluid (CSF) reservoir and prevent the fluid from flowing back to the brain, decreasing the pressure and fluid level in the brain to normal levels.

A is incorrect because lumbar puncture is not a treatment for hydrocephalus. A lumbar puncture is used to collect a sterile sample of CSF for laboratory testing, relieve pressure, inject dye, or inject medication.

B is incorrect because osmotic diuretics are not a treatment for hydrocephalus.

D is incorrect because monitoring intracranial pressure is an important nursing assessment but is not a treatment for hydrocephalus.

15. A 6-month-old infant is admitted to the neurological unit for hydrocephalus. Which of the following does the nurse expect to find when assessing the infant?

    A. Normal growth and development
    B. Enlarged head circumference
    C. Infant is able to sit upright unassisted
    D. Unresponsiveness

Rationale:

Correct answer: B

Hydrocephalus is accumulation of the spinal fluid within the brain due to abnormal production or recycling of the fluid in the neurological system. This leads to rapid enlargement of the head and neurological disruption. Symptoms of hydrocephalus include enlargement of head circumference, nystagmus, convulsions, vomiting, irritability, delay of growth and meeting developmental milestones, and failure to thrive. Other common findings with hydrocephalus include a prominent forehead, dilated scalp veins, and widened, tense fontanelles.

A is incorrect because children with hydrocephalus tend to have delayed growth and development.

C is incorrect because the 6-month-old infant with hydrocephalus is usually unable to sit upright unassisted due to developmental delay.

D is incorrect because hydrocephalus may cause somnolence but does not cause unresponsiveness.

16. The mother of an infant admitted with cerebral palsy is upset about the child's diagnosis. She explains that she experienced a normal pregnancy and delivery. When the mother asks what she did to cause this, what is the best response by the nurse?

    A. "Your child's cerebral palsy may be due to your ingestion of sushi during pregnancy."
    B. "The cerebral palsy is due to complications during delivery."
    C. "It's not always known why cerebral palsy occurs, but it happens during development of the baby's brain."
    D. "Cerebral palsy is usually due to jaundice at birth."

Rationale:

Correct answer: C

Cerebral palsy affects function of the brain and nervous system and includes several different types. The etiology of cerebral palsy is not always clear, but is possibly due to brain bleed, encephalitis or meningitis, head injury, or rubella infection in the mother during pregnancy.

A is incorrect because ingestion of sushi during pregnancy is not linked to increased incidences of cerebral palsy. Brain damage and hearing and vision problems have been linked to maternal ingestion of sushi and other mercury-containing foods during the prenatal period.

B is incorrect because some cases of cerebral palsy are related to a traumatic delivery, anoxia during birth, or infection at the time of delivery, but the mother already indicated that the pregnancy and delivery were uncomplicated. The nurse should use caution making definitive, accusatory, presumptive statements.

D is incorrect because jaundice develops after birth and would have to be severe in order to increase the risk of cerebral palsy.

17. The nurse on the pediatric ward is caring for a 4-year-old female patient with spastic cerebral palsy. When observing the child ambulating, which of the following does the nurse expect to see?

    A. Tight muscles and abnormal gait
    B. Seizure activity
    C. Muscle weakness and hypermobile joints
    D. Increased muscle mass in lower extremities

Rationale:

Correct answer: A

Cerebral palsy is a group of permanent disorders that affect function of the brain and development of the child's nervous system. Movement and posture are affected, causing activity limitation due to disturbances that occurred in the developing fetal or infant brain. Spastic cerebral palsy, the most common type of cerebral palsy, is characterized by symptoms including tight muscles and abnormal gait, joint contracture, and paralysis in groups of muscles.

B is incorrect because although the risk for seizures is increased with cerebral palsy in general, seizure activity is not expected when assessing the gait of a child with spastic cerebral palsy.

C is incorrect because although muscles weakness may be seen, hypermobility of joints is not expected with spastic cerebral palsy. Joint contractures are more common.

D is incorrect because children with cerebral palsy often have decreased muscle mass.

18. The parents of a 9-year-old girl diagnosed with attention deficit hyperactivity disorder (ADHD) ask the nurse what they can do to help their child. Which of the following suggestions does the nurse make?

A. Speak with her teacher about putting her in a large class with other children the same age
B. Provide lenient rules and be patient
C. Praise her for good behavior and give rewards
D. Avoid schedules and routines to decrease the child's frustration

Rationale:

Correct answer: C

ADHD is a collection of one or more symptoms related to focus, activity, and control of behavior. Children with ADHD will be inattentive, hyperactive, or impulsive, or any combination of the three symptoms. Helping the child with ADHD consists of regularly speaking with the teacher, small class size, setting consistent rules, praising good behavior, maintaining normal schedules and routines, providing for sufficient sleep, and limiting distractions.

A is incorrect because, although children with ADHD can often thrive in a classroom with others of the same age group and developmental stage, they benefit from a small class size.

B is incorrect because the parent of a child with ADHD should be encouraged to use both consistency and patience when enforcing rules.

D is incorrect because the child with ADHD benefits from regular schedules and routines.

19. The nurse in the family practice clinic is teaching the parents of an 8-year-old boy with attention deficit hyperactivity disorder (ADHD) regarding a new prescription for dextroamphetamine. When the parents ask how the medication works, what is the best response by the nurse?

A. "The medication will increase your child's mental alertness to help him focus in school."

B. “The medication will help your child sleep better at night.”
C. “Monitor your child’s heart rate when starting this medication, as it can cause the heart to beat more slowly.”
D. “This medication will decrease motor activity, so your child won’t fidget as much.”

Rationale:

Correct answer: A

ADHD is a collection of one or more symptoms related to focus, activity, and control of behavior. Dextroamphetamine is a CNS stimulant that facilitates the release of catecholamines which increases motor activity, enhances mental alertness, and decreases drowsiness to help the child focus.

B is incorrect because the medication is a stimulant which can cause insomnia, so it should be given in the morning.

C is incorrect because the medication is a stimulant which can cause tachycardia and palpations.

D is incorrect because the medication stimulates the nervous system and increases motor activity. Fidgeting is a common side effect with administration of this type of drug.

20. The parents of a 4-year-old girl have brought their child to the family practice clinic to be evaluated for changes in mobility. The parents report that she has started tripping and falling, has become very clumsy, complains of leg pain, and is no longer able to climb stairs at home. Which of the following does the nurse suspect?

A. Hydrocephaly
B. Myelomeningocele
C. Cerebral palsy

D. Muscular dystrophy

Rationale:

Correct answer: D

Muscular dystrophy is an inherited, terminal muscular disorder that causes progressive muscle weakness, atrophy, and replacement with fatty tissue over time. The nerves are not affected. Symptoms include clumsy movements, difficulty with stair climbing, tripping and falling frequently, leg pain, and weakness. Diagnosis usually occurs between the ages of 3 and 6 years. Treatment includes intense physical therapy, frequent range of motion, and often, the use of leg braces to help with ambulation.

A is incorrect because the symptoms are not characteristic of hydrocephaly. Hydrocephaly is an accumulation of cerebrospinal fluid in the brain, and common symptoms in a pre-school-aged child are high-pitched cry, changes in personality, crossed eyes, difficulty feeding, sleepiness, headache, and irritability.

B is incorrect because myelomeningocele is a type of spina bifida in which the unfused portion of the spinal column allows the spinal cord to protrude through an opening. This diagnosis is either made while the fetus is in utero, or shortly after birth, not at age 4.

C is incorrect because cerebral palsy symptoms are present at birth, and do not suddenly worsen at the age of 4.

21. A 12-year-old girl is admitted to the emergency room following a fall off of a horse. She is disoriented and restless and determined to have sustained a concussion. Which of the following nursing diagnoses is the highest priority?

    A. Disturbed visual sensory perception
    B. Self-care deficit

C. Impaired verbal communication
D. Risk for injury

Rationale:

Correct answer: D

A concussion is a traumatic injury of the brain that jars the brain within the skull. There are usually no visible signs of brain injury with a concussion, and symptoms include losing consciousness, inability to remember what happened, repetitive questions, confusion, disorientation, and restlessness. The patient is at risk for injury due to disorientation and restlessness. The nurse should keep the patient's bed in the lowest position, raise side rails to prevent falling from the bed, and monitor the patient closely.

A is incorrect because disturbed visual sensory perception may be present with a concussion but is not a greater priority than physical safety.

B is incorrect because no information is provided to indicate that the child is experiencing a self-care deficit.

C is incorrect because the information given about the patient does not indicate that the child is having difficulty with verbal communication and this is not a greater priority than physical safety from injury.

22. The nurse is caring for a 15-year-old patient with paraplegia at the T4 level due to a history of a skateboarding accident which occurred nine months ago. Which of the following interventions should the nurse perform to prevent autonomic dysreflexia in this patient?

    A. Support a high-protein diet
    B. Discuss sexuality and fertility options
    C. Plan a bowel program
    D. Teach quad coughing

Rationale:

Correct answer: C

Autonomic dysreflexia is uncontrolled hypertension with acute onset that can develop in patients with spinal cord injury at the level of T6 and above. It can lead to seizures, pulmonary edema, myocardial infarction, hemorrhage, and death. A common stimulus is fecal impaction (due to the patient's inability to sense the need to have a bowel movement), so a bowel program should be planned to prevent impaction from developing. Other causes of autonomic dysreflexia include bladder distention, pain, and tactile stimulation. Nursing priorities include emptying the urinary bladder frequently (patient self-catheterization or straight-catheterization by the nurse) and that linens are not creased underneath the patient.

A is incorrect because a high-protein diet will not prevent fecal impaction or autonomic dysreflexia. The diet should contain adequate fiber and liquids to keep stool soft and minimize the likelihood of constipation or impaction.

B is incorrect because discussion of sexuality and fertility options is not appropriate for a 15-year-old and will not prevent autonomic dysreflexia.

D is incorrect because, although teaching coughing and incentive spirometry exercises are important for respiratory health, these will not prevent autonomic dysreflexia.

23. A 5-year-old girl is scheduled for magnetic resonance imaging (MRI). Which of the following actions should be implemented by the nurse before the test?

   A. NPO status for 12 hours prior to the MRI
   B. Withhold all daily medications until after the MRI is completed
   C. Administer morphine for prevention of claustrophobia
   D. Place the patient in gown with cloth ties

Rationale:

Correct answer: D

MRI has a magnetic field, and metal objects are a hazard around the MRI. A gown with cloth ties should be placed on the patient to prevent injury to the patient. If a gown with metal snaps is used, this can cause burning to the skin.

A is incorrect because if a child requires sedation for an MRI, NPO status is generally required for eight hours prior to the procedure.

B is incorrect because withholding daily medications may not be necessary for an MRI.

C is incorrect because morphine is an opiate pain medication which is not used to prevent claustrophobia during an MRI. If the child has a history of claustrophobia or experiences claustrophobia during the procedure, anxiolytic medications may be administered.

24. The nurse is caring for a 6-year-old patient with Guillain-Barre syndrome. Which of the following actions is most important?

  A. Treatment of peripheral pain with acetaminophen
  B. Encourage the child to participate in activities of daily living
  C. Determine if the child has recently been ill
  D. Assessment of progression of muscle weakness

Rationale:

Correct answer: D

Guillain-Barre is an autoimmune disorder which leads to the immune system attacking nerves, which causes patients to be temporarily paralyzed over time. Early symptoms include sensation changes with pain and muscle weakness beginning in the feet and hands and progressing up the legs and arms. This weakness can spread to respiratory muscles and may require mechanical ventilation. Assessing the progression of muscle weakness and respiratory effort is the greatest priority.

A is incorrect because Guillain-Barre can cause pain, but assessment of muscle weakness is the greater physical priority.

B is incorrect because it is beneficial to the child to participate in ADLs as tolerated, but assessment of respiratory status and muscle weakness is the greater concern.

C is incorrect because Guillain-Barre can be triggered by recent infection, but determining the cause is not more important than current physical assessment.

25. A nurse on the pediatric neurological unit performs a neurological assessment on an unresponsive 11-year-old boy. When painful stimuli are introduced, the boy's arms are drawn up to the middle of the chest with the elbows bent and backs of the hands together, and the toes are pointed inward. How does the nurse document the finding?

    A. Decorticate posturing
    B. Decerebrate posturing
    C. Atypical hyperreflexia
    D. Glasgow Coma Scale (GCS) motor response score: 4

Rationale:

Correct answer: A

Decorticate posturing occurs when there is an interruption of the corticospinal pathway. The arms are flexed with the backs of the hands pressed together in the middle of the chest, and toes are pointed toward the midline. This is an abnormal finding and is indicative of brain damage. The healthcare provider must be notified immediately when this occurs.

B is incorrect because decerebrate posturing is external rotation and extension of extremities, and this type of posturing is indicative of more severe brain damage, often involving the brainstem.

C is incorrect because hyperreflexia is increased reflex response.

D is incorrect because a GCS motor response score of 4 is documented if the child withdraws to painful stimuli. Decorticate posturing scores a motor response score of 3.

CHAPTER 4:

NCLEX-RN – PEDIATRIC CARDIOVASCULAR - 25 QUESTIONS

1. The nurse is talking with the parents of a 6-week-old infant regarding their child's cardiac catheterization for repair of a ventricular septal defect (VSD) and home care. Which of the following instructions does the nurse include in the discharge teaching?

   A. "Restrict the child's physical activity for 2 weeks following the procedure."
   B. "The incision cannot be submerged in water, so give the child a sponge bath daily until the stitches are removed."
   C. "Prophylactic antibiotics must be used before future dental procedures."
   D. "Keep the pressure dressing on the site until the healthcare provider evaluates it."

Rationale:

Correct answer: C

A Ventricular Septal Defect (VSD) occurs when the hole between the ventricles of the heart does not close before the fetus is born. This allows blood between the ventricles to mix, which decreases oxygenation of the blood. A VSD repair closes the hole in the septum between the ventricles. The surgeon sews the hole closed or patches the hole with the baby's own tissue or a synthetic patch. Patients with heart defects must have prophylactic antibiotics before any future dental procedures to reduce the risk of infection.

A is incorrect because activities do not need to be restricted after a VSD repair.

B is incorrect because stitches are not used after cardiac catheterization.

D is incorrect because a pressure dressing is not used after discharge for cardiac catheterization. The parents will be taught how to change the clean dressing at home and inspect the puncture site for signs of infection.

2. A 2-year-old girl diagnosed with Tetralogy of Fallot is having blood drawn for routine tests when she becomes upset, turns blue, and her breathing rate increases to 46 breaths per minute. Which intervention does the nurse perform first?

    A. Contact the healthcare provider for a sedation order
    B. Assess the child's heart rate and rhythm for irregularity
    C. Reassure the child that mild pain is expected during the blood draw
    D. Position the child with knees to chest

Rationale:

Correct answer: D

Tetralogy of Fallot is a congenital heart defect that includes ventricular septal defect, pulmonary stenosis, hypertrophy of the right ventricle, and an overriding aorta. The knees-to-chest position will reduce venous return, thereby reducing shunting of blood through the defect in the septum, which increases oxygen in the systemic blood circulation and decreases dyspnea and tachypnea.

A is incorrect because sedation is not needed unless repositioning is ineffective.

B is incorrect because further assessment should be performed after repositioning the child. The knee to chest position will most immediately help with the child's breathing.

C is incorrect because reassuring the child is an appropriate psychosocial intervention, but this will not relieve the hypoxia. The nurse must prioritize actual physical needs over psychosocial needs.

3. A 6-year-old is admitted to the pediatric emergency room with rheumatic fever. When assessing the child, which of the following signs does the nurse identify as an initial sign of infective endocarditis?

   A. Anterior chest wall pain
   B. Irregular heart rhythm
   C. Heart murmur
   D. Hypotension

Rationale:

Correct answer: C

Rheumatic fever typically develops 2 to 4 weeks after a strep throat infection. Infective endocarditis occurs when the bacteria enter the bloodstream and settle in the heart lining, a heart valve or a blood vessel, causing infection and inflammation of the endocardium. With endocarditis, heart murmurs can present in approximately 75 percent of patients in the first week. Other symptoms include fever and chills, aching joints, night sweats, and fatigue.

A is incorrect because anterior chest wall pain does not usually occur with infective endocarditis. This type of pain is commonly a sign of costochondritis, an inflammation of costochondral junctions of ribs or chondrosternal joints of the anterior chest wall.

B is incorrect because the heart rhythm with endocarditis is commonly tachycardia but is not irregular.

D is incorrect because hypotension does not usually occur with endocarditis.

4. A 12-year-old boy with a history of asthma visits the school nurse reporting chest pain. After the nurse confirms that the boy has not had complications with his asthma in several years, what is the next action the nurse should perform?

   A. Obtain peak flow reading
   B. Instruct the boy to lay down for 10 minutes
   C. Call the child's parents for more information
   D. Administer two puffs of a short-acting bronchodilator

Rationale:

Correct answer: A

Asthma is chronic inflammation and obstruction in the lungs with symptoms including chest tightness, wheezing, coughing, and shortness of breath. More assessment needs to be done before intervening with this child. A peak flow reading and vital signs should be obtained before notifying the parents or healthcare provider.

B is incorrect because the priority is assessing the airway. Having the boy lie down may make it more difficult for him to breathe.

C is incorrect because immediate airway assessment needs to be performed before notifying the parents.

D is incorrect because assessment needs to be performed before administering a short-acting bronchodilator. The nurse must obtain a baseline measurement using the peak flow meter to determine if the bronchodilator is necessary.

5. A 7-year-old girl with a history of asthma tells the school nurse she is interested in joining one of the school's sports teams. Which of the following sports does the nurse suggest for her?

   A. Soccer
   B. Track and field
   C. Swimming
   D. Ice skating

Rationale:

Correct answer: C

Asthma is chronic inflammation and obstruction in the lungs with symptoms including chest tightness, wheezing, coughing, and shortness of breath. Swimming is a low-impact sport that promotes ventilation and perfusion while enhancing skeletal muscle mass. Any sport that requires frequent stop-and-start exertion can cause asthma exacerbation. Sports suggested for asthmatic children include swimming, baseball or softball, golf, martial arts, fencing, and volleyball.

A is incorrect because soccer is a vigorous activity which takes place over a long period of time and can cause asthma exacerbation.

B is incorrect because track and field often involves a level of intensity that can be hard on the respiratory system and cause asthma exacerbation.

D is incorrect because cold-weather activities, such as ice skating, ice hockey, snow skiing, or snowboarding, can be hard on asthma sufferers. They're taxing on the lungs and on the body.

6. The nurse is teaching the parents of a 6-year-old with cystic fibrosis (CF) regarding dietary choices. Which of the following is not an appropriate food choice for the child?

   A. Roasted pork tenderloin
   B. Fried chicken
   C. Skim chocolate milkshake
   D. Egg omelet

   Rationale:

   Correct answer: B

   Cystic fibrosis (CF) affects production of mucous and sweat, causing dysfunction in the lungs and digestive system. CF children have a deficiency of pancreatic enzymes, disrupting the body's ability to digest and absorb fat, leading to weight loss. Patients with cystic fibrosis require a high-nutrient, high-protein, and low-fat diet with pancreatic enzyme replacement.

   A is incorrect because roasted pork tenderloin is nutrient and protein dense.

   C is incorrect because a skim milkshake is low in fat and offers a good source of calories.

   D is incorrect because an egg omelet is nutrient dense.

7. The nurse is caring for infants in the intensive care unit (ICU). Which of the following is at the greatest risk for sudden infant death syndrome (SIDS)?

   A. 3-month-old infant who is laid to sleep on his back
   B. 6-month-old infant who has had pneumonia twice
   C. First born infant of a 40-year-old mother
   D. 2 month old with frequent 5-second apnea episodes

Rationale:

Correct answer: D

Sudden infant death syndrome (SIDS) is unexplained and sudden death of a child under the age of 1 year. Infants between the ages of 2 and 4 months have the highest risk of SIDS, and apnea episodes greater than 20 seconds indicate a higher risk of SIDS. Other factors that increase the risk for SIDS include when the baby gets too hot during sleep, shares a bed with others, sleeps on soft surfaces (such as an adult mattress), or sleeps under soft or loose bedding.

A is incorrect because lying the baby on his back to sleep is safe. When a baby sleeps on his stomach, the risk for SIDS increases.

B is incorrect because respiratory illness does not increase risk of SIDS.

C is incorrect because older maternal age does not increase risk of SIDS.

8. The nurse finds a 4-year-old boy unresponsive and not breathing in the daycare center. After instructing another individual to call 911, which of the following interventions does the nurse perform next?

   A. Give a precordial thump
   B. Give breaths with bag-valve-mask (BVM) at a rate of 16 bpm
   C. Open and clear the airway
   D. Start chest compressions at a rate of 100 per minute

Rationale:

Correct answer: C

Clearing the airway is always the first intervention in cardiopulmonary resuscitation, especially when the collapse was not witnessed. In children, apnea and unconsciousness are usually due to pathophysiology of the respiratory system. Time is very important when dealing with an unconscious child who is not breathing. Permanent brain damage begins after only 4 minutes without oxygen, and death can occur as soon as 4 to 6 minutes later.

A is incorrect because a precordial thump is generally not indicated for pediatrics. This medical procedure is used in the treatment of ventricular fibrillation or pulseless ventricular tachycardia in those with witnessed, monitored onset of one of the "shockable" cardiac rhythms if a defibrillator is not immediately available. It should not be used in those with unwitnessed or out-of-hospital cardiac arrest.

B is incorrect because the airway should be cleared before giving breaths.

D is incorrect because in incidences where the nurse did not witness the collapse, the airway should be cleared, and rescue breaths should be given before compressions are started. (If the nurse witnessed the child suddenly collapse, rescue breaths should be skipped, and compressions should be started.)

9. The nurse in the pediatric cardiac unit is caring for a 2-year-old scheduled for heart surgery. Which of the following interventions does the nurse use to best decrease anxiety for the child's parents?

   A. Reassure the parents of the surgeon's success rate
   B. Offer to obtain an order for an anxiolytic for the parents
   C. Teach the parents and the child about the surgery one month before the surgery
   D. Explain the steps involved before and after the procedure

Rationale:

Correct answer: D

Heart surgery in pediatrics is performed to correct congenital heart defects. It is appropriate for the nurse to give the parents something tangible to focus on by explaining what to expect. This is often an effective way to reduce the parents' anxiety about the upcoming procedure and enable them to cooperate in the plan of care.

A is incorrect because the nurse needs to hear the concerns of the parents instead of dismissing them by focusing on the surgeon.

B is incorrect because obtaining anxiolytics for the parents is inappropriate. The parents are not the patient.

C is incorrect because preoperative teaching should be performed within a week of the surgery, not one month.

10. The nurse in the pediatric cardiac unit is caring for a 3-year-old child with Kawasaki disease. The nurse knows which of the following medications is typically administered to children with Kawasaki disease?

    A. Acetaminophen
    B. Amoxicillin
    C. Aspirin
    D. Ibuprofen

Rationale:

Correct answer: C

Kawasaki disease is an autoimmune disease often seen in children under the age of 5 years. The disease causes vasculitis that affects small- and medium-sized blood vessels and lymph nodes and may progress to affect the patient's coronary arteries. Aspirin is administered daily to children with Kawasaki disease for anti-inflammatory purposes as well as to control fever. Once fever subsides, aspirin is continued as an antiplatelet. Immunoglobulins are also administered in the initial treatment for Kawasaki.

A is incorrect because acetaminophen does not have blood-thinning properties and is often ineffective in reducing the fever in a child with Kawasaki.

B is incorrect because amoxicillin is not effective for treating Kawasaki. Amoxicillin is an antibiotic which can be used to treat a bacterial infection. (Kawasaki is an autoimmune disease, which can be triggered by infection.)

D is incorrect because the blood-thinning properties of ibuprofen are not as effective as aspirin.

11. The nurse in the neonatal intensive care unit (NICU) is assessing a 1-week-old male infant. When the brachial, radial, and femoral pulses are palpated, a difference in amplitude is noted between the bilateral femoral and radial pulses. The nurse knows this finding suggests which of the following?

    A. Patent ductus arteriosus
    B. Coarctation of the aorta
    C. Increased cardiac output
    D. Fluid volume overload

Rationale:

Correct answer: B

Coarctation of the aorta is narrowing of the aorta below the left subclavian artery. This requires the left ventricle to generate a much higher pressure than normal in order to force enough blood through the aorta to deliver blood to the lower part of the body. If the left ventricle is not strong enough to push blood through the narrowed aorta, the result may be decreased blood flow to the lower half of the body, which can cause a difference in amplitude between the femoral and radial pulses (in which the radial pulse is generally stronger than the femoral pulse bilaterally). Coarctation is twice as common in boys than in girls.

A is incorrect because patent ductus arteriosus (PDA) is manifested by bounding pulse due to left-to-right shunting of the blood in the heart. Irregular transmission of blood from the aorta to the pulmonary artery occurs. Other symptoms include tachycardia, dyspnea, and poor growth. PDA has a high occurrence in premature newborns.

C is incorrect because increased cardiac output is manifested by a strong and bounding pulse, not a difference between femoral and radial pulses.

D is incorrect because fluid volume overload in a newborn would be characterized by weight gain, edema, a bounding pulse, shortness of breath, and pulmonary congestion.

12. The nurse in the pediatric cardiac unit is caring for a 3-year-old boy diagnosed with Tetralogy of Fallot. When the nurse assesses the boy, the nurse expects fatigue and poor activity tolerance, which are caused by which of the following?

    A. Poor muscle tone
    B. Inadequate oxygenation of tissues
    C. Restriction of blood flow leaving the heart
    D. Inadequate intake of food

Rationale:

Correct answer: B

Tetralogy of Fallot is a cyanotic congenital heart defect which includes four defects: ventricular septal defect, pulmonary stenosis, hypertrophy of the right ventricle, and an overriding aorta. The condition causes left-to-right shunting of the blood in the heart which causes inadequate oxygenation of tissues.

A is incorrect because poor muscle tone is a result of Tetralogy of Fallot, not a cause. Other findings of Tetralogy of Fallot include clubbing of the fingers, poor sucking reflex, lethargy, and cyanosis.

C is incorrect because restriction of blood flow leaving the heart is caused by aortic stenosis, which is a narrowing of the aortic valve that decreases cardiac output.

D is incorrect because Tetralogy of Fallot causes a poor sucking reflex and lethargy, which results in inadequate food intake. However, the *cause* is poor tissue oxygenation due to mixed blood between the right and left sides of the heart.

13. The nursing student in the pediatric cardiac unit is learning about congenital heart defects. The student learns that which congenital heart defect causes pediatric cyanosis?

    A. Atrial septal defect
    B. Coarctation of the aorta
    C. Ventricular septal defect
    D. Transposition of the great vessels

Rationale:

Correct answer: D

Transposition of the great vessels means the pulmonary artery is connected to the left ventricle and the aorta is connected to the right ventricle, causing blood to reach the tissues before being oxygenated in the lungs. This leads to cyanosis in the pediatric patient.

A is incorrect because an atrial septal defect (abnormal opening between the right and left atria of the heart) is an acyanotic congenital malformation.

B is incorrect because coarctation of the aorta narrows the aorta and decreases oxygenated blood circulation to the body. Coarctation is an acyanotic congenital malformation.

C is incorrect because ventricular septal defect (abnormal opening between the right and left ventricles of the heart) is an acyanotic congenital malformation.

14. The nurse in the pediatric intensive care unit (PICU) is caring for a 6-week-old female patient diagnosed with Tetralogy of Fallot (TOF). When assessing the child, the nurse expects to find which common physiologic adaptation?

    A. Clubbing of the fingers
    B. Slow, irregular respirations
    C. Subcutaneous hemorrhage
    D. Decreased red blood cell count

Rationale:

Correct answer: A

TOF is a congenital heart defect that includes ventricular septal defect, pulmonary stenosis, hypertrophy of the right ventricle, and an overriding aorta. Symptoms include bluish color to the skin and clubbing of the fingers due to hypoxia causing poor circulation to the periphery. When the infant cries or has a bowel movement, they may experience a "tet" spell in which the child turns very blue in color, has difficulty breathing, becomes limp, and may even lose consciousness. Other symptoms may include a heart murmur and fatigue when feeding.

B is incorrect because TOF is characterized by shortness of breath, not slow and irregular respirations.

C is incorrect because subcutaneous hemorrhage is not commonly seen with TOF. Subcutaneous hemorrhage in infants is usually the result of birth trauma or certain rare viruses.

D is incorrect because TOF does not cause an abnormally low number of red blood cells. A compensatory mechanism for the cyanotic congenital heart defects is polycythemia, or increased hemoglobin and/or red blood cells.

15. The nurse in the pediatric cardiac unit is caring for a 5-year-old boy diagnosed with a ventricular septal defect (VSD) who is scheduled for a cardiac catheterization. The nurse tells the boy's parents the purpose of the cardiac catheterization is:

    A. To identify the specific location of the VSD
    B. To determine the degree of cardiomegaly
    C. To confirm the presence of a pansystolic murmur
    D. To establish the presence of ventricular hypertrophy

Rationale:

Correct answer: A

Ventricular septal defect (VSD) is an acyanotic congenital heart defect. This occurs when the hole between the ventricles of the heart does not close before the fetus is born, allowing blood between the ventricles to mix, which decreases oxygenation of the blood pumped out of the heart. The size can vary from as small as a pin-hole to the child having no septum at all. The purpose of cardiac catheterization with VSD is to determine the specific location and size of the defect and to assess pressures in the pulmonary system.

B is incorrect because cardiomegaly is determined by echocardiogram, not catheterization.

C is incorrect because a pansystolic murmur (also known as a harsh holosystolic murmur, heard at the left lower sternal border) can generally be detected by cardiac auscultation with a stethoscope and does not require catheterization to be detected. This is the classic murmur heard in patients with VSD.

D is incorrect because although ventricular hypertrophy is common with VSD, it is not determined by catheterization.

16. The nurse in the pediatric clinic is assessing a 5-year-old girl with a congenital cardiac defect. When the mother asks why her daughter squats after exertion, the nurse tells the mother this position does which of the following?

    A. Reduces muscle aches
    B. Increases cardiac efficiency
    C. Relieves anxiety associated with high blood pressure
    D. Decreases blood volume in the extremities

Rationale:

Correct answer: B

Congenital heart defects are abnormalities of the heart that develop in utero or failure of normal in-utero shunts to close before or during birth. Squatting causes blood to pool in the lower extremities due to flexion of the hips and knees. This causes a decrease in blood volume returning to the heart, which allows the heart to beat more effectively.

A is incorrect because the squatting position after physical exertion is not due to aching muscles, it is a result of dyspnea.

C is incorrect because squatting does not directly relieve anxiety, and children with congenital heart defects do not squat because of abnormal blood pressure; they assume this position because of breathlessness after exertion.

D is incorrect because the squatting position retains blood volume in the extremities which improves efficiency of the cardiac pump.

17. An infant diagnosed with Tetralogy of Fallot becomes cyanotic and dyspneic following an episode of crying. For relief of the cyanosis and dyspnea, the nurse places the infant in which position?

    A. Orthopneic position
    B. Knee-chest position
    C. Lateral Sims' position
    D. Semi-fowler's position

Rationale:

Correct answer: B

Tetralogy of Fallot (TOF) is a congenital heart defect that includes ventricular septal defect, pulmonary stenosis, hypertrophy of the right ventricle, and an overriding aorta. Flexing the knees and hips will decrease venous blood return to the heart from the extremities, which will decrease the workload of the heart.

A is incorrect because the orthopneic position is a position in which the patient assumes an upright or semi-vertical position by using pillows to support the head and chest or sits upright in a chair. This is used for people who have difficulty breathing when lying down but is not associated with relief of dyspnea from TOF.

C is incorrect because the lateral Sims' position is generally used for rectal treatment, enema, or examination. The patient lies on the left side with the left hip and lower extremity straight and right hip and knee bent.

D is incorrect because a Semi-fowler's position (laying supine with the head of bed elevated at 30 to 45 degrees) does not help relieve the dyspnea associated with TOF after a crying episode (or physical exertion).

18. The nurse in the neonatal cardiac unit is caring for a 2-week-old patient diagnosed with congenital heart disease and heart failure. The nurse knows the most appropriate action is which of the following?

    A. Positioning the infant prone after feeding
    B. Encouraging PO water intake
    C. Offering small, frequent feedings
    D. Measuring head circumference

Rationale:

Correct answer: C

Congenital heart defects are abnormalities of the heart that develop in utero or failure of normal in utero shunts to close before or during birth. Congenital heart disease with heart failure causes extreme fatigue with sucking in an infant, so smaller, frequent feedings and adequate rest periods should be provided to improve nutritional intake.

A is incorrect because positioning a child with congenital heart disease and heart failure prone after feeding is unsafe. The baby should be placed on its right side after feeding to prevent the risk for aspiration.

B is incorrect because an infant at the age of 2 weeks does not need PO water.

D is incorrect because assessment of head circumference is not a specific priority assessment of a newborn with congenital heart disease and heart failure.

19. An 8-year-old female patient is admitted to the pediatric cardiac unit with myocarditis and tachycardia. The healthcare provider has ordered furosemide to be administered every 12 hours. Which of the following lab values does the nurse closely monitor?

   A. Calcium
   B. Glucose
   C. Potassium
   D. Sodium

Rationale:

Correct answer: C

Myocarditis is inflammation of the heart muscle, and tachycardia is increased heart rate for patient age. Furosemide is a loop diuretic that rids the body of excess fluid but also wastes potassium. The potassium level should be monitored frequently for the duration of the time that the child is receiving furosemide. If symptoms of hypokalemia are present, the nurse should hold the next dose of furosemide and check the potassium level before administering the medication.

A is incorrect because monitoring of calcium is not necessary with furosemide.

B is incorrect because monitoring of glucose is not necessary with furosemide.

D is incorrect because monitoring of sodium is not necessary with furosemide.

20. The nurse in the pediatric cardiac intensive care unit (ICU) is caring for a 1-month-old female patient who has been admitted for confirmation of ventricular septal defect. When assessing the infant, the nurse expects to find which of the following?

A. Bradycardia at rest
B. Bounding upper extremity peripheral pulses
C. Activity related cyanosis
D. Murmur at left sternal border

Rationale:

Correct answer: D

Ventricular septal defect (VSD) occurs when the hole between the ventricles of the heart does not close before the fetus is born, allowing blood between the ventricles to mix and decreasing oxygenation of the blood. A loud, harsh murmur at the left sternal border is an expected finding in a child with VSD.

A is incorrect because pediatric bradycardia at rest is characteristic of AV block, not VSD.

B is incorrect because bounding upper extremity peripheral pulses are characteristic of coarctation of the aorta, not VSD.

C is incorrect because activity-related cyanosis is characteristic of Tetralogy of Fallot, not VSD.

21. The nurse in the pediatric unit is providing discharge instructions to the parents of a 4-year-old boy with Tetralogy of Fallot. When teaching the parents about hypercyanotic spells ("tet spells"), the nurse tells the parents they should:

    A. Call the healthcare provider immediately
    B. Use a calm, comforting approach
    C. Lay the child supine
    D. Take the child to the emergency room

Rationale:

Correct answer: B

Tetralogy of Fallot (TOF) is a congenital heart defect that includes ventricular septal defect, pulmonary stenosis, hypertrophy of the right ventricle, and an overriding aorta. In TOF, hypercyanotic spells ("tet spells") result in extreme bluish discoloration of mucous membranes and skin. Parents must maintain a calm and comforting approach and place the child in the knee-to-chest position, which will help relieve the dyspnea.

A is incorrect because notifying the healthcare provider is not the first action for the parents to take. A calm approach is helpful in relieving the dyspnea the child is experiencing, and proper positioning of the child is the priority. The healthcare provider will assess frequency of "tet" spells at regular clinic visits.

C is incorrect because the supine position is not the proper position for reducing cardiac workload associated with "tet" spells in TOF.

D is incorrect because taking the child to the emergency room is not necessary unless profound hypoxia occurs after proper positioning.

22. A 3-month-old infant has been prescribed digoxin to be given at home for chronic tachyarrhythmia. When teaching the mother about digoxin, which of the following statements is appropriate for the nurse to include?

    A. "Be sure to report blurred vision to the healthcare provider immediately."
    B. "You can expect your baby's heart rate to be elevated while taking this medication."
    C. "Vomiting for two or more feedings may be a sign of toxicity and should be reported immediately."

D. “Bulging of the anterior fontanel may be a sign that the digoxin level is too low.”

Rationale:

Correct answer: C

Signs of digoxin toxicity include blurred vision, yellow-green visual spots, nausea, and vomiting, but only objective symptoms such as vomiting can be assessed by the mother of a 3-month-old.

A is incorrect because blurred vision cannot be assessed in a 3-month-old patient.

B is incorrect because digoxin decreases the heart rate.

D is incorrect because bulging of the anterior fontanel (which indicates increased intracranial pressure) is not related to administration of digoxin to an infant.

23. The nurse is caring for a 2-year-old who is recovering from cardiac catheterization for diagnosis of a congenital heart defect. When assessing the child, which of the following indicates immediate action by the nurse is warranted?

A. Decreased pulse
B. Decreased urine output
C. Respirations 34 per minute
D. Bleeding from catheter site

Rationale:

Correct answer: D

Cardiac catheterization is performed in pediatric patients to locate and identify abnormalities of the heart. Bleeding from the catheter site could become threatening and warrants immediate action by the nurse. Pressure should be applied to the site immediately.

A is incorrect because the greatest concern after a cardiac catheterization is hemorrhage, which would present with increased pulse, not decreased.

B is incorrect because decreased urine output should be further assessed, but urine output is not a greater concern than potential hemorrhage. This finding could be due to the child lying supine during and after the catheterization.

C is incorrect because the normal respiratory rate for a toddler is 20 to 40 per minute.

24. The nurse is caring for a 9-year-old boy admitted for myocarditis experiencing tachycardia. The healthcare provider has prescribed digoxin. Before administering the digoxin, the nurse must assess which of the following?

    A. Apical pulse
    B. Urine output
    C. Bilateral pulse equality
    D. Blood pressure

Rationale:

Correct answer: A

Digoxin is a cardiac glycoside medication that is administered to decrease heart rate and improve myocardial contractility. This drug should not be administered if the child's is bradycardic. The most accurate method of measuring heart rate in a child is assessing the apical pulse. Normal pulse for a 9-year-old is 60 to 95 beats per minute.

B is incorrect because urine output assessment is not a priority before administering digoxin.

C is incorrect because pulse equality assessment is not a priority before administering digoxin to a child.

D is incorrect because blood pressure assessment is not necessary before administering digoxin.

25. The nurse in the pediatric intensive care unit (PICU) is assessing a 5-year-old boy admitted with heart failure. The boy weighs 40 lbs. When assessing the child, which of the following indicates adequate cardiac output?

    A. Urine output 30 mL/hr
    B. Heart rate 120 bpm
    C. Capillary refill 6 to 7 seconds
    D. Bilateral crackles heard on auscultation

Rationale:

Correct answer: A

Heart failure is inability of the heart to pump effectively, causing the backing up of blood within the cardiovascular system, which can lead to edema and decrease urine output. Minimal hourly urine output should be 1-2 mL/kg/hr. in children. This child weighs 40 lbs.=18.14 kg. Normal urine output for this child should be 18-36mL/hr., so 30 mL/hr. indicates the heart is pumping effectively and cardiac output is adequate.

B is incorrect because a 5-year-old's heart rate should be between 60 and 95 bpm. Tachycardia suggests the heart is having to beat faster than normal to maintain adequate perfusion throughout the body. This is an indication that cardiac output is not adequate.

C is incorrect because capillary refill should be less than 2 seconds. Delayed capillary refill indicates decreased cardiac output.

D is incorrect because crackles are abnormal and could indicate worsening heart failure or hypervolemia.

CHAPTER 5:

NCLEX-RN - PEDIATRIC: RESPIRATORY – 25 QUESTIONS

1. A 9-year-old boy who is blind and developmentally delayed must be assisted with all meals. The boy has difficulty with swallowing and frequently coughs and chokes with feedings. The nurse should feed this child using which technique?

   A. Hold the child upright and use a soft tip bulb syringe
   B. Place the child supine and turn the boy's head to the right
   C. Prop the child semi-sitting, chop up food, and place it in the boy's mouth with a plastic utensil
   D. Seat the boy in a wheelchair, give small bites with metal utensils, and encourage the child to participate

Rationale:

Correct answer: D

Seating a patient in an upright position will help prevent aspiration. Metal utensils are safer than plastic as they will not break. Socializing with the child enhances the nurse-client relationship. Encouraging participation enhances the child's likelihood in interacting with the staff and engaging in his own care.

A is incorrect because a soft tip bulb syringe is not appropriate for feeding a 9-year-old child.

B is incorrect because placing the child supine during mealtimes will increase the risk for aspiration.

C is incorrect because the child does not have an infectious process that requires the use of disposable utensils. Furthermore, plastic utensils can break, increasing the risk for injury during feeding.

2. An 8-year-old boy goes to see the school nurse complaining of difficulty breathing. What is the first action the nurse should perform?

   A. Take vital signs
   B. Call the boy's mother
   C. Administer an aerosol treatment
   D. Listen to the boy's lungs

Rationale:

Correct answer: D

Difficulty breathing in a school-age child is commonly due to an asthma attack. Immediate assessment of the lungs is the priority before intervening. The priority is to gather a baseline assessment of the ability of the lungs to move air, so the nurse can reassess after intervening. Further respiratory assessment for shortness of breath, wheezing, and coughing should also be performed.

A is incorrect because vital signs are not the first action the nurse should take. The child is displaying signs of respiratory distress, so the respiratory system assessment is the greatest concern.

B is incorrect because calling the mother is not the first action. The nurse should remain on the physical care of the boy, here-and-now.

C is incorrect because the lungs must be assessed before administration of an aerosol treatment.

3. An 11-year-old girl with a history of asthma is diagnosed with status asthmaticus in the emergency room. The nurse knows that this means the child:

   A. Has severe wheezing
   B. Hasn't responded to treatment
   C. Requires an emergency tracheostomy
   D. Has underlying pneumonia

   Rationale:

   Correct answer: B

   Status asthmaticus is asthma with moderate-to-severe airway obstruction that does not respond to initial treatment; there is no improvement in the asthma when treatments are administered.

   A is incorrect because wheezing stops with status asthmaticus as airways are obstructed. (Severe wheezing precedes status asthmaticus.)

   C is incorrect because intubation may not be needed with status asthmaticus. If so, oral intubation would be attempted before a tracheostomy.

   D is incorrect because pneumonia and status asthmaticus are not related.

4. The nurse is admitting a 16-month-old to the pediatric respiratory unit with a diagnosis of croup. The nurse is most concerned by which of the following?

   A. Inspiratory stridor is heard
   B. The mother is unable to calm the child
   C. The toddler has a barking cough

D. The toddler has a decreased appetite

Rationale:

Correct answer: B

Croup is a respiratory problem that commonly occurs in young children in the fall and winter months. Croup will cause swelling and narrowing of the airway, causing a harsh, barking cough, and leads to dyspnea. If the mother is unable to calm the child, the nurse should assess for worsening hypoxia.

A is incorrect because inspiratory stridor (whistling noise heard upon inspiration) is common with croup and is not an indication of a complication.

C is incorrect because a barking cough is a common and expected finding with a diagnosis of croup.

D is incorrect because children often have a decreased appetite when ill.

5. A 2-year-old with severe croup is admitted to the pediatric intensive care unit (PICU) and oxygen is administered via nasal cannula. The nurse knows oxygen is administered for which purpose?

   A. It congeals mucous secretions and relieves dyspnea
   B. It decreases effort of breathing and allows for rest
   C. It triggers cough reflex and facilitates mucous expectoration
   D. It decreases the child's anxiety related to hypoxia

Rationale:

Correct answer: B

Croup is a respiratory problem that commonly occurs in young children in the fall and winter months. Croup will cause swelling and narrowing of the airway, causing a harsh, barking cough, and leading to dyspnea.

Supplemental oxygen via nasal cannula helps meet the child's oxygen needs and thus decreases the effort of breathing, allowing the child to rest and conserve energy for nutritional and fluid intake.

A is incorrect because croup does not cause mucous secretions, and oxygen therapy does not have a direct effect on the viscosity of respiratory secretions.

C is incorrect because mucous expectoration is not an effect of oxygen therapy, and secretions are not common with croup.

D is incorrect because the main purpose of oxygen therapy is to increase oxygen circulating in the blood, not to decrease anxiety. (Hypoxia may cause anxiety, but the relieving anxiety is not the primary purpose of the supplemental oxygen.)

6. A 3-year-old in the pediatric intensive care unit (PICU) is admitted for streptococcal pneumonia and hypoxia. When the child is intubated with an oral endotracheal (ET) tube, which outcome indicates successful intubation?

   A. Bilateral breath sounds heard on auscultation
   B. SpO_2 88%
   C. Audible cry heard on inspiration
   D. Chest X-ray shows the tip of ET tube is in right mainstem bronchus

Rationale:

Correct answer: A

Streptococcal pneumonia is pneumonia caused by streptococcus bacteria and causes dyspnea, decreased oxygenation, and atelectasis. Intubation is insertion of an artificial airway (oral ET tube) for improved oxygenation and support of the airway. Intubation is successful when bilateral breath sounds are heard on auscultation and the oxygen level in the blood (measured by pulse oximetry or arterial blood gas) returns to normal.

B is incorrect because the pulse-oximeter reading (SpO_2) should be higher after intubation. (Normal SpO_2 is 95-100%.)

C is incorrect because no cries should be heard when oral intubation is successful, as the cuff is inflated, and the child should not be able to make vocal sounds.

D is incorrect because intubating the right mainstem bronchus will not fully oxygenate the child.

7. A 4-year-old boy is brought to the pediatric emergency room, and the parents report he recently swallowed a small toy. Which of the following symptoms suggest the airway is completely obstructed by a foreign body?

   A. Gagging
   B. Coughing
   C. Inability to speak
   D. Rapid respirations, client's hands are placed over his throat

Rationale:

Correct answer: C

Complete airway obstruction causes inability to cough, breath, or speak. If the child is unable to cough or speak, the airway is completely obstructed and requires emergency intervention.

A is incorrect because gagging is due to laryngotracheal obstruction but is not an indication of partial or full blockage.

B is incorrect because coughing requires the movement of air and confirms that the airway is only partially occluded.

D is incorrect because rapid respirations are expected with partial airway obstruction and do not indicate complete airway obstruction. Patients with a foreign object in the airway will often place their hands over their throat, but this does not confirm complete airway blockage.

8. A 5-year-old girl is brought to the pediatric emergency room displaying drooling, strident cough, and lethargy. The healthcare provider suspects epiglottitis. What is the priority intervention for this child?

   A. Take vital signs
   B. Prepare for intubation
   C. Visualize the child's throat with tongue depressor
   D. Obtain throat cultures

Rationale:

Correct answer: B

This child has classis signs of epiglottitis, or inflammation of the epiglottis, which is a medical emergency in pediatric patients. The nurse must prepare for intubation to secure the airway.

A is incorrect because assessment of vital signs needs to be completed, but the airway is the priority.

C is incorrect because visualizing the child's throat does not confirm epiglottitis and is not a priority assessment at this time. Enough assessment data is already present to know that the child needs help breathing.

D is incorrect because throat cultures are performed to determine the causative agent in an infectious process but do not address the airway at this time.

9. A 7-year-old boy is one-day post-operative tonsillectomy. When the child vomits coffee-ground-like material, what is the most appropriate action by the nurse?

   A. Notify the healthcare provider immediately
   B. Maintain NPO status for 24 hours
   C. Maintain NPO for 30 minutes, then try clear liquids
   D. Place the child supine

Rationale:

Correct answer: C

Tonsillectomy is a procedure performed to remove the tonsils due to recurrent tonsillitis, airway obstruction, or debris (tonsil stones). Vomit that resembles coffee grounds is old blood, which is common after tonsillectomy. The child should be NPO for 30 minutes, then clear liquids resumed, and the nurse should assess for active bleeding. (Bright red fluid at the back of the throat, hypotension, and tachycardia indicate active bleeding.)

A is incorrect because notification of the healthcare provider is not necessary unless the child is experiencing active bleeding.

B is incorrect because NPO for 24 hours is not necessary.

D is incorrect because the child should be prone or side-lying for prevention of aspiration.

10. A 7-year-old in the emergency room is experiencing an acute asthma attack. Which medication should the nurse prepare to administer?

   A. Terbutaline
   B. Beclomethasone dipropionate
   C. Prednisone
   D. Albuterol

Rationale:

Correct answer: D

Asthma is characterized by narrowing and obstruction of the alveoli, causing dyspnea, coughing, and wheezing. Albuterol is a beta-2 adrenergic agonist that causes bronchodilation, which is a rescue bronchodilator indicated for an acute asthma attack.

A is incorrect because terbutaline is indicated for long-term control of asthma.

B is incorrect because beclomethasone dipropionate is indicated for long-term control of asthma.

C is incorrect because prednisone is a steroid medication which is used for 3 to 10 days after an acute asthma attack.

11. An 8-year-old boy admitted for status asthmaticus appears to be improving. The best method of evaluating response to therapy is for the nurse to:

    A. Auscultate breath sounds
    B. Monitor respiratory pattern
    C. Assess lips for decreased cyanosis
    D. Evaluate current peak expiratory flow rate

Rationale:

Correct answer: D

Status asthmaticus is asthma with moderate-to-severe airway obstruction that does not respond to initial treatment. A peak expiratory flow meter measures the maximum volume of air flow that can be forcefully exhaled in one second and is compared to the individualized personal best value. This comparison is the most effective way to determine the current respiratory status.

A is incorrect because breath sounds are not the best method of evaluating response to therapy.

B is incorrect because monitoring respiratory pattern is not the best method of evaluating response to therapy.

C is incorrect because cyanosis is a late sign of respiratory distress and may take some time to resolve. Resolution of cyanosis is not an accurate way to determine current oxygenation status.

12. A 5-year-old child is in the pediatric medical-surgical unit following surgery. The child is drowsy and not following commands. In order to maintain the child's airway, the nurse should perform which intervention?

    A. Have a tongue blade available
    B. Keep the child supine and immobilize the cervical spine
    C. Use nasotracheal suction every 8 to 10 minutes
    D. Place the child in lateral Sims' position

Rationale:

Correct answer: D

Lateral Sims' position allows fluids to drain from the mouth and prevents aspiration while the child is still drowsy from anesthesia.

A is incorrect because a tongue blade can be used to open the mouth but does not maintain the child's airway.

B is incorrect because supine position could increase the risk for aspiration, and the child does not need cervical spine immobilization.

C is incorrect because nasotracheal suction is used in the post-anesthesia unit and should not be needed in the medical-surgical unit unless the patient has excessive amounts of respiratory secretions.

13. A 7-year-old girl rescued from a house fire the previous day is in the pediatric intensive care unit with burns to the upper arms and back of the neck. Smoke inhalation has led to a deterioration in the child's respiratory condition. Which of the following should the nurse be alert for?

    A. Infection
    B. Tracheobronchial edema
    C. Posttraumatic stress disorder
    D. Generalized adaptations to stress

Rationale:

Correct answer: B

Any burns sustained to the upper extremities, head, face, neck, trunk, or upper back increase the risk for airway compromise. Heat and smoke inhalation can cause fluid to shift from the intravascular compartment into the interstitial compartment, which results in edema and obstructs the airway. This can be delayed for 24 to 48 hours.

A is incorrect because smoke inhalation does not directly cause infection.

C is incorrect because posttraumatic stress disorder does not occur 24 hours after an incident.

D is incorrect because generalized adaptations to stress do not occur 24 hours after an incident.

14. A child with cystic fibrosis is in the clinic with early signs of an upper respiratory tract infection with a moderate cough and a runny nose. The nurse teaches the child's mother to do which of the following?

    A. Make sure the child eats well
    B. Take the child's temperature twice per day

C. Offer plenty of orange juice
D. Increase chest physiotherapy to four times daily

Rationale:

Correct answer: D

Cystic fibrosis affects production of mucous and sweat, causing dysfunction in the lungs and digestive system. An upper respiratory tract infection could develop into pneumonia for this child if secretions aren't loosened and removed with percussion and postural drainage.

A is incorrect because eating well is important to maintain optimal nutritional intake, but chest physiotherapy is the priority.

B is incorrect because monitoring the child's temperature is important to determine if the infection is worsening, but chest physiotherapy is important because it can help prevent the worsening of infection.

C is incorrect because orange juice is important but not as much as chest physiotherapy.

15. The nurse in the pediatric medical-surgical unit is caring for a 10-year-old girl with cystic fibrosis. The child tells the nurse she feels like she isn't getting enough air. Which of the following indicates compensation for decreased blood oxygen levels?

    A. Sunken abdomen
    B. Distended jugular veins
    C. Edema in lower extremities
    D. Clubbing of fingers and toes

Rationale:

Correct answer: D

Cystic fibrosis affects production of mucous and sweat, causing dysfunction in the lungs and digestive system. Clubbing of fingers and toes indicates collateral circulation has been built to compensate for decreased oxygen levels.

A is incorrect because a sunken abdomen is an indication of malnutrition or infection with a parasite.

B is incorrect because distended jugular veins indicate circulatory volume overload or superior vena cava syndrome.

C is incorrect because lower extremity edema can be a manifestation of several different disorders, including heart failure, kidney disease, liver cirrhosis, or as a result of mechanical ventilation.

16. The nurse in the pediatric medical-surgical unit is caring for a 12-year-old female with cystic fibrosis. When reviewing the medication record, the nurse notes a dose of pancreatic enzymes is due this morning. When should the nurse administer the medication?

    A. With breakfast
    B. After breakfast
    C. With antibiotics
    D. 2 hours before breakfast

Rationale

Correct answer: A

Cystic fibrosis (CF) affects production of mucous and sweat, causing dysfunction in the lungs and digestive system. Supplemental pancreatic enzymes help the CF patient digest dietary fat and should be administered with high-calorie, high-protein meals for breakdown of dietary fat and increased absorption.

B is incorrect because pancreatic enzymes should be administered with meals.

C is incorrect because pancreatic enzymes should be administered with meals, and PO antibiotics should be taken 1 hour before or 2 hours after meals to maximize antibiotic absorption.

D is incorrect because administration of pancreatic enzymes 2 hours before a meal will not achieve the full effect for maximizing fat absorption during meal digestion.

17. The nurse is caring for a 6-month-old admitted for bronchiolitis. Which of the following is an important nursing measure for this infant?

    A. Promote stimulating activities that meet the infant's developmental needs
    B. Make regular assessments of the infant's skin color, anterior fontanel, and vital signs
    C. Discourage parental visits during the acute phase for conservation of the infant's energy
    D. Maintain airborne precautions including donning a gown, cap, mask, and gloves when providing care

Rationale:

Correct answer: B

Bronchiolitis is inflammation, infection. and congestion of the bronchioles (the small air passageways in the lungs) caused by a virus, commonly respiratory syncytial virus (RSV). Bronchiolitis typically lasts 2 to 3 weeks and the child can typically be cared for at home. When hospitalized, assessments of skin color, anterior fontanel, and vital signs are important for monitoring of hydration and oxygenation status.

A is incorrect because stimulating activities may increase the demand for energy and leave the child with less energy for breathing.

C is incorrect because energy must be conserved, but parents should be encouraged to visit their infant in a calm and restful environment.

D is incorrect because airborne precautions are not necessary with bronchiolitis.

18. A 6-month-old infant is admitted with bronchiolitis and respiratory syncytial virus (RSV). The nurse places the infant in a private room and institutes which type of precautions?

    A. Droplet
    B. Standard
    C. Contact
    D. Airborne

Rationale:

Correct answer: C

Bronchiolitis is inflammation of the bronchioles caused by a virus, commonly respiratory syncytial virus (RSV). Although this is usually treated at home, when a child is hospitalized for RSV, contact precautions should be initiated as the virus can live on surfaces for up to 6 hours. Clean gloves are to be worn for contact with the patient or the patient's belongings or surfaces in the patient's room. Gloves must be removed before leaving the client's environment, and hands must be washed with an antimicrobial soap. A gown must be worn if the nurse is going to come into contact with the patient or contaminated items in the patient's environment.

A is incorrect because droplet precautions are not necessary with RSV. Examples of diseases that require droplet precautions include diphtheria, group *A. streptococcus* pneumonia, *H. influenza* type B, rubella, mumps, and pertussis.

B is incorrect because contact precautions are used with RSV, in addition to standard precautions.

D is incorrect because airborne precautions are not necessary with RSV. Airborne precautions are required for varicella, tuberculosis, measles, and disseminated zoster.

19. The mother of a 3-year-old boy calls the nurse into the hospital room and says her son is choking. What is the priority intervention by the nurse?

    A. Open the child's mouth and sweep for foreign material
    B. Give five back blows with the child over the nurse's arm face down
    C. Assess whether the child can make vocal sounds
    D. Perform five subdiaphragmatic abdominal thrusts with the child supine

Rationale:

Correct answer: C

Complete airway obstruction causes inability to cough, breath, or speak. If the child is unable to speak, the airway is completely obstructed and requires emergency intervention. Thus, the nurse's initial priority action is to determine if the airway is fully obstructed. (If the child is able to cough or speak, the nurse should encourage the child to continue coughing until the object becomes dislodged or it becomes evident that the airway has become fully obstructed.)

A is incorrect because performing a blind sweep can push a foreign object further into the airway and cause obstruction.

B is incorrect because back blows in this position are used on children age 1 year or younger.

D is incorrect because abdominal thrusts are performed after confirmation of complete airway obstruction.

20. The nurse is caring for a 6-month-old girl admitted with bronchiolitis. The nurse organizes care to allow for uninterrupted periods of rest. This plan is:

   A. Inappropriate because constant care is necessary in the acute phase of bronchiolitis
   B. Appropriate because cool mist helps maintain hydration status
   C. Inappropriate because frequent assessment by auscultation is required
   D. Appropriate because this promotes decreased oxygen demands

Rationale

Correct answer: D

Bronchiolitis is inflammation of the bronchioles caused by a virus, commonly respiratory syncytial virus (RSV). Allowing periods of uninterrupted rest promotes decreased oxygen demands.

A is incorrect because constant care increases oxygen needs.

B is incorrect because cool mist helps humidify the airway but does not maintain hydration status or meet the child's fluid needs.

C is incorrect because frequent airway assessment by auscultation increases oxygen needs. It is appropriate to cluster care in order to provide adequate rest time, as the child with bronchiolitis is often fatigued. The nurse should assess the airway every 2 hours and as needed if the child's condition deteriorates.

21. A 12-year-old boy with a history of asthma visits the school nurse reporting chest pain. When the nurse determines the boy has not had problems with his asthma in several years, what is the next action the nurse should perform?

   A. Obtain a peak flow reading

B. Instruct the boy to lie down for 30 minutes
C. Call the child's parents for more information
D. Administer two puffs of the child's short-acting bronchodilator

Rationale:

Correct answer: A

Asthma is chronic inflammation and obstruction in the lungs with symptoms including chest tightness, wheezing, coughing, and shortness of breath. More assessment needs to be done before intervening with this child. A peak flow reading will indicate how compromised the airways are and will help the nurse determine which course of action to take next. This critical assessment is necessary before administering medications, notifying the parents, or contacting the healthcare provider.

B is incorrect because further airway assessment needs to be performed before having the boy change position. An elevated head of bed facilitates easier breathing, so if the airways are constricted, assuming a lying down position will not help.

C is incorrect because calling the parents for information does not give pertinent information about the airway and current respiratory status.

D is incorrect because assessment needs to be performed before administering a short-acting bronchodilator. A baseline respiratory assessment must be done to determine how constricted the airways are so the nurse can re-evaluate after administration of a medication.

22. The nursing student in the family clinic is learning about respiratory infections in children. The nursing student learns that infants younger than 3 months of age have better resistance to respiratory infections due to:

A. Frequent checkups

B. Maternal antibodies
C. Inability to breathe through their nose
D. Lack of exposure

Rationale:

Correct answer: B

While in utero, the developing fetus acquires maternal antibodies that protect the infant at birth and for up to 3 months after birth. This decreases the risk of respiratory infections in infants.

A is incorrect because frequent checkups do not prevent respiratory infections.

C is incorrect because nose-breathing does not prevent respiratory infections.

D is incorrect because infants are still potentially exposed to respiratory infections by coming into contact with people in the home, siblings, people in the community, or other children at daycare.

23. The nurse is assessing a newborn in the family clinic, and the mother tells the nurse the infant has been having difficulty nursing. The nurse knows newborns can have difficulty breathing while nursing if:

A. They have developed colic
B. The mother is obese
C. The environment is too warm
D. The nares are not patent

Rationale

Correct answer: D

Infants up to 4 weeks of age are nose breathers and are unable to breathe through their mouths. If for any reason the nares are not patent, such as mucus or underdeveloped nares, the newborn will be unable to breathe while nursing, which can affect nutritional status.

A is incorrect because colic does not affect breathing while nursing.

B is incorrect because maternal weight does not affect breathing while nursing unless the mother's breasts are so large that they occlude the infant's nostrils.

C is incorrect because environmental temperature does not affect breathing while nursing.

24. An 8-year-old boy is brought to the emergency room by his parents complaining that "he seems to be breathing fast." When the nurse assesses the boy, no fever is present, the respiratory rate is 35 bpm, and he has a nonproductive cough. The parents report the child recently had a cold. Which of the following is an appropriate statement by the nurse?

  A. Acute asthma
  B. Bronchial pneumonia
  C. Chronic obstructive pulmonary disease (COPD)
  D. Emphysema

Rationale

Correct answer: A

Asthma is chronic inflammation and obstruction in the lungs with symptoms including chest tightness, wheezing, coughing, and shortness of breath. Due to the child's history and symptoms, acute asthma is most likely the diagnosis.

B is incorrect because bronchial pneumonia in children is characterized by a productive cough and elevated temperature.

C is incorrect because COPD does not typically occur in children. (COPD is most prevalent in older and middle-aged adults but is not a normal part of aging.)

D is incorrect because emphysema does not occur in children. Emphysema is the over-inflation of the alveoli. Predisposing factors include smoking, environmental pollution, and chronic infections.

25. An 8-year-old with acute asthma is in the emergency room displaying inspiratory and expiratory wheezes and decreased expiratory volume. Which of the following classes of medications does the nurse anticipate administering?

    A. Beta-adrenergic blockers
    B. Bronchodilators
    C. Inhaled steroids
    D. Oral steroids

Rationale

Correct answer: B

Asthma is chronic inflammation and obstruction in the lungs with symptoms including chest tightness, wheezing, coughing, and shortness of breath. Bronchodilators are considered first-line treatment due to the bronchoconstriction that occurs with asthma, which reduces airflow.

A is incorrect because beta-adrenergic blockers are not used in asthma. These medications are used to control hypertension and to treat angina and migraines.

C is incorrect because inhaled steroids are not for emergency relief in asthma.

D is incorrect because oral steroids are not for emergency relief in asthma.

CHAPTER 6:

NCLEX-RN – PEDIATRIC: GI METABOLIC ENDOCRINE - 25 QUESTIONS

1. The nurse in the pediatric medical-surgical unit is caring for a 9-year-old child admitted with diabetes insipidus. Which of the following signs does the nurse recognize as characteristic of diabetes insipidus?

   A. Weight gain
   B. Increased urine specific gravity
   C. Increased urination
   D. Serum sodium 130 mEq/L

   Rationale:

   Correct answer: C

   Diabetes insipidus is due to a deficiency of antidiuretic hormone, which causes increased urinary output and fluid loss. This can lead to dehydration, hypernatremia, excessive thirst, weakness, and constipation. Causes of diabetes insipidus include head trauma, brain injury, meningitis, or encephalitis.

A is incorrect because diabetes insipidus causes fluid loss, which causes weight loss.

B is incorrect because increased urine specific gravity is due to concentrated urine or syndrome of inappropriate antidiuretic hormone (SIADH).

D is incorrect because diabetes insipidus leads to increased serum sodium concentration, or greater than 145 mEq/L.

2. The parent of a 6-year-old diagnosed with diabetes mellitus asks why self-monitoring of blood glucose is recommended. What knowledge does the nurse base the explanation on?

   A. It is less expensive
   B. It is more accurate than lab testing
   C. Parents and children are better able to manage the diabetes
   D. Frequent self-monitoring can slow the progression of the disease

Rationale:

Correct answer: C

Diabetes is a condition of lack of insulin or insulin resistance that increases blood sugar levels. Data collected through frequent self-monitoring of blood sugar helps the child and parents to determine how different activities and foods affect blood sugar levels. The child and parents can then better manage the diabetes by adjusting insulin dosage based on results of the blood sugar tests.

A is incorrect because blood glucose monitoring is more expensive but provides improved management.

B is incorrect because self-monitoring is equivalent to lab testing. Most home glucose meters on the market today measure glucose from plasma, which is the same way blood glucose is measured in the clinical setting.

D is incorrect because self-monitoring allows for better diabetes control but does not directly slow progression or prevent complications of the disease. For example, peripheral neuropathy is a late complication of diabetes that tends to occur after an individual suffers from diabetes for many years, but blood glucose monitoring does not prevent this type of complication or progression.

3. A 10-year-old girl with diabetes type 1 is in the clinic for an upper respiratory infection. Her parents report she is not eating and ask the nurse what action is best. What is the best recommendation by the nurse?

   A. Give her half of her morning dose of insulin
   B. Substitute simple carbohydrates or liquids with calories for solid food
   C. Allow plenty of unsweetened, clear liquids for prevention of dehydration
   D. Take her to the emergency room immediately

Rationale:

Correct answer: B

Diabetes type 1 is a condition of lack of insulin production in the islet cells of the pancreas, leading to increased blood sugar. Diabetic "sick day rules" apply whenever a patient with diabetes is ill, overly stressed, or sick. A "sick day diet" of simple carbohydrates or liquids with calories will maintain normal blood sugar levels and decrease the risk of hypoglycemia. Other "sick day rules" include taking the normally ordered dose of insulin or oral antidiabetic agent, checking blood glucose every 3 to 4 hours, checking urine for ketones, and eating small meals frequently.

A is incorrect because the child should receive the regular dose of insulin, despite decreased appetite.

C is incorrect because calories are needed to prevent hypoglycemia.

D is incorrect because diabetes and minor illnesses such as a respiratory infection can be managed safely at home. The healthcare provider should be contacted to report abnormal blood glucose, fever, vomiting, or diarrhea.

4. A 12-year-old boy is admitted to the pediatric medical-surgical unit for suspected hypothyroidism. Which of the following is a common clinical manifestation of juvenile hypothyroidism?

   A. Insomnia
   B. Diarrhea
   C. Dry skin
   D. Accelerated growth

Rationale:

Correct answer: C

Hypothyroidism is decreased thyroid activity including decreased production of thyroid hormones. Manifestations include dry skin, mental decline, constipation, cold intolerance, and weight gain.

A is incorrect because hypothyroidism causes sleepiness. Insomnia is a symptom of hyperactive thyroid.

B is incorrect because diarrhea is a symptom of hyperthyroidism. Hypothyroidism causes constipation.

D is incorrect because decelerated growth and development occurs in children with hypothyroidism.

5. The nurse in the pediatric unit is caring for a child admitted to investigate potential growth hormone deficiency. When discussing possible metabolic alterations with the parents, which of the following should the nurse include?

   A. Hypercalcemia
   B. Hypoglycemia
   C. Diabetes insipidus
   D. Hyperglycemia

   Rationale:

   Correct answer: B

   Growth hormone stimulates growth of internal body organs and assists in maintaining normal blood sugar levels. Growth hormone deficiency can lead to hypoglycemia.

   A is incorrect because hypercalcemia is associated with hyperparathyroidism.

   C is incorrect because diabetes insipidus is due to posterior pituitary disorder. Growth hormone deficiency, in rare cases, can lead to type 2 diabetes mellitus.

   D is incorrect because hyperglycemia is due to lack of insulin.

6. The nurse in the pediatric medical-surgical unit is caring for a 14-year-old boy admitted with Graves' disease. When planning care, which of the following is a priority nursing goal for this adolescent?

   A. Encouraging adequate fluid intake to relieve constipation
   B. Allowing the adolescent to make decisions regarding taking his medications
   C. Verbalizing the importance of medication regimen adherence
   D. Developing alternative educational plans

Rationale:

Correct answer: C

Graves' disease is an auto-immune disorder and the leading cause of hyperactivity of the thyroid gland. The medication regimen includes taking specific medications, sometimes two to three times each day. The adolescent must understand the importance of adherence to the medication regimen and verbalize intent to comply.

A is incorrect because a patient with Graves' disease does need adequate fluids to prevent dehydration from diarrhea but not to relieve constipation.

B is incorrect because although it is appropriate to encourage the adolescent patient to take an active role in his care, decisions about medications should not be made by the individual. The priority regarding medications is to teach the adolescent about compliance with the medication schedule and not to skip or alter doses.

D is incorrect because managing Graves' disease does not require alternative educational plans. Adolescents place a high priority on social interaction with peers. The patient should be encouraged to continue attending school and social events as well as participating in athletic and leisure activities, despite a diagnosis of Graves' disease (which is non-debilitating and non-contagious).

7. A 6-year-old girl is in the clinic with her parents for precocious puberty. Which of the following is the most appropriate intervention for the child?

   A. Prepare age-appropriate educational materials regarding the use of birth control for the child
   B. Explain the importance of having the child develop relationships with her peers

C. Reassure the parents that the risk for sexual abuse is not increased due to her appearance
D. Counsel the parents that there is no treatment currently for precocious puberty

Rationale:

Correct answer: B

Precocious puberty is early onset of secondary sex characteristics in young children. (Puberty onset before the age of 9 in girls is considered "early.") The child needs to be treated according to her chronologic age and interact with peers of the same age group to encourage age-appropriate behavior and social interactions.

A is incorrect because birth control is not appropriate for a 6-year-old and will not delay precocious puberty. Gonadotropin-releasing hormone blocker medications can be administered to delay the progression of puberty. The parents should also be counseled about how to appropriately talk to the child about how her body is changing.

C is incorrect because research shows that there is an increased risk for sexual abuse due to precocious puberty.

D is incorrect because gonadotropin-releasing hormone blocker is administered for precocious puberty.

8. A 10-year-old boy recently diagnosed with growth hormone (GH) deficiency is beginning treatment with GH. Which of the following instructions does the nurse give the parents regarding administration of the GH injections?

A. Encourage the boy to give himself the injection at bedtime
B. Administer the injection to the child after meals
C. Give the medication before meals after checking blood glucose

D. Encourage the boy to administer his GH injection on arising in the morning, before breakfast

Rationale:

Correct answer: A

Growth hormone injection treatment is prescribed for children who have been diagnosed with growth hormone (GH) deficiency and other conditions causing short stature. Because natural growth hormone is released mainly during sleep in children, GH treatment is more effective when injections are given at bedtime in order to closely approximate the normal physiologic release of GH. Children age 10 and older should be encouraged to participate in their own care by learning how to give themselves the injections under the supervision of an adult to ensure proper dosage and injection technique. Self-injection has been shown to increase children's self-esteem and to feel some sense of control of their care.

B is incorrect because after meals does not closely approximate physiologic release of GH, and the child should be encouraged to give himself the injections.

C is incorrect because GH injections are given at bedtime, not before meals, and do not require checking blood glucose before administration.

D is incorrect because giving GH in the morning does not closely approximate physiologic nocturnal release of GH.

9. A 3-day-old neonate with ambiguous genitalia is diagnosed with congenital adrenogenital hyperplasia. Which of the medications does the nurse anticipate administering?

A. Vitamin D

B. Cortisone

C. Stool softeners

D. Calcium carbonate

Rationale:

Correct answer: B

Congenital adrenogenital hyperplasia is a genetic condition that prevents the adrenal glands from producing certain enzymes involved in the synthesis of cortisol or aldosterone, or both. This affects growth and development in children. The nurse would anticipate administering cortisone due to this hormone deficiency. Additionally, the nurse would anticipate a blood karyotype test in the infant with ambiguous genitalia to establish the chromosomal sex.

A is incorrect because vitamin D is not part of congenital adrenogenital hyperplasia treatment. Vitamin D supplementation is encouraged for breastfed newborns who may not receive enough sun exposure to stimulate the body's own production of vitamin D.

C is incorrect because stool softeners are not part of congenital adrenogenital hyperplasia treatment. Stool softeners should be used very cautiously in newborns, as they can lead to diarrhea and dehydration.

D is incorrect because calcium carbonate is not part of congenital adrenogenital hyperplasia treatment. In children, calcium carbonate is most often used to treat a calcium deficiency.

10. The parents of a newborn in the family clinic ask the nurse why the infant needs blood tests. What is the best response by the nurse regarding priority outcomes of mandatory newborn screening for metabolic disorders?

    A. "The tests are performed so we can make appropriate community referrals."

B. “This helps us provide education regarding raising a special needs child.”
C. “The test assists with early identification of genetically transmitted metabolic diseases.”
D. “It helps us with early identification of electrolyte imbalances.”

Rationale:

Correct answer: C

Newborns are routinely screened with blood testing for metabolic disorders such as phenylketonuria, congenital hypothyroidism, and congenital adrenal hyperplasia. Infants with these disorders may not show symptoms until it’s too late to provide adequate treatment, thus the need for early detection in mandatory newborn blood screenings.

A is incorrect because community referrals are not made until after a specific diagnosis is made.

B is incorrect because education is not the primary goal of mandatory screening.

D is incorrect because electrolyte imbalances are not metabolic disorders and are not the priority outcome assessed with newborn screening.

11. The nurse in the pediatric unit is caring for children with metabolic and endocrine disorders. Which of the following endocrine disorders can cause exophthalmos?

A. Hypothyroidism
B. Hyperthyroidism
C. Hypoparathyroidism
D. Hyperparathyroidism

Rationale

Correct answer: B

Exophthalmos is protrusion of the eyeballs, which is sometimes seen with hyperthyroidism. Other more serious causes of exophthalmos in children include acute intracranial hypertension, rhabdomyosarcoma, and neuroblastoma.

A is incorrect because hypothyroidism does not cause exophthalmos. Hypothyroidism causes weight gain, fatigue, constipation, and delayed growth in children.

C is incorrect because hypoparathyroidism does not cause exophthalmos. Hypoparathyroidism causes imbalances in calcium and phosphorus levels.

D is incorrect because hyperparathyroidism does not cause exophthalmos. Hyperparathyroidism causes too much calcium in the blood and a deficiency of calcium in the bones, leading to bone fragility in children, among other vaguer symptoms.

12. A 3-month-old is admitted to the pediatric intensive care unit for hypertrophic pyloric stenosis after several days of vomiting. Which of the following nursing diagnoses is priority?

    A. Deficient fluid volume related to prolonged vomiting
    B. Ineffective airway clearance related to impaired swallowing
    C. Imbalanced nutrition: less than body requirements related to prolonged vomiting
    D. Anxiety related to loss of body control

Rationale:

Correct answer: A

Hypertrophic pyloric stenosis is obstruction of the gastric outlet due to hypertrophy and hyperplasia of the pylorus, which is the most common cause of vomiting in infants. Dehydration is common in infants with pyloric stenosis, due to the large amount of fluid ingested that does not reach the small intestine for proper absorption. Replacement of fluids and electrolytes is priority.

B is incorrect because swallowing is not affected by pyloric stenosis. The infant with acute pyloric stenosis is at risk for aspiration but does not necessarily have the inability to clear the airway.

C is incorrect because imbalanced nutrition is an appropriate nursing diagnosis but not a greater priority than fluid status.

D is incorrect because infants do not typically experience anxiety related to body control. (Even if infant anxiety was present, this would be a psychosocial concern, which would not be a greater priority than fluid balance, which is a greater physical need.)

13. The nurse in the family practice clinic is interviewing the mother of an infant who has suspected intussusception. Which of the following questions does the nurse ask to obtain the most useful history?

    A. "Is your child eating normally?"
    B. "How often has your child been vomiting?"
    C. "What do your infant's stools look like?"
    D. "When did your child last urinate?"

Rationale:

Correct answer: C

Intussusception is invagination of the intestines into adjoining intestinal lumen (usually the ileum into the cecum and colon) which causes bowel obstruction and blocked blood and lymph circulation. It is a medical emergency which requires surgical intervention to repair the defect. Stools commonly look like currant jelly because of mucus, inflammation, and hemorrhage in the bowel. The diagnosis can often be made on assessment of the infant's behavior and stool alone. Other symptoms include a tender, distended abdomen, the child drawing their knees up to their abdomen, and vomiting. Sometimes a sausage-shaped mass can be palpated in the upper right abdominal quadrant. Intussusception is most commonly seen in children ages 3-months to 3-years.

A is incorrect because feeding history is not as relevant to intussusception as stool appearance.

B is incorrect because vomiting history is not specific to intussusception.

D is incorrect because urination history is not relevant to intussusception.

14. The healthcare provider has reduced an infant's hernia and schedules the herniorrhaphy in two days. When the parents ask why the procedure is delayed, what is the best response by the nurse?

    A. "Delaying the procedure ensures proper preparations are made with the surgical team."
    B. "Delaying the procedure allows swelling and inflammation in the area to subside."
    C. "Surgery cannot be attempted unless your infant has worn a truss for 48 hours."
    D. "We must make sure your child has nothing to eat or drink for 8 to 12 hours before the surgery."

Rationale:

Correct answer: B

Hernia is protrusion of a section of intestine through a weak spot in the abdominal wall, and herniorrhaphy is surgical repair of a hernia. Swelling and inflammation occur after reduction of a hernia, and risk of complications decreases when surgery is delayed, allowing time for the inflammation to decrease.

A is incorrect because the delay between hernia reduction and repair is not for the purpose of preparation.

C is incorrect because the infant does not need to wear a truss.

D is incorrect because NPO status in infants is generally required for 3 to 6 hours before surgery, depending on the surgeon's orders.

15. The nurse in the family practice clinic is assessing an infant diagnosed with Hirschsprung's disease. Which of the following does the nurse expect to find?

    A. Scaphoid abdomen
    B. Cyanosis of distal extremities
    C. Hyperactive reflexes
    D. Weight less than normal for height and age

Rationale:

Correct answer: D

Hirschsprung's disease is a disease of the large intestine that interferes with the passage of stool due to nerve cells in the colon missing at birth. Failure to thrive is common in children with Hirschsprung's disease, and due to malabsorption of nutrients, children weigh less than normal. Symptoms include failure to pass meconium, refusal to suck, and abdominal distention.

A is incorrect because the abdomen is distended in Hirschsprung's disease.

B is incorrect because cyanosis is related to congenital heart disease.

C is incorrect because infant hyperreflexia can reflect epilepsy or other central nervous system disorder but is not related to Hirschsprung's disease.

16. An 18-lb., 8-month-old infant is admitted to the emergency room for severe diarrhea. Which of the following findings would alert the nurse to notify the healthcare provider?

    A. Hyperactive bowel sounds
    B. Depressed anterior fontanel
    C. 72 mL pale yellow urine over the past four hours
    D. Absence of tenting during skin turgor assessment

Rationale:

Correct answer: B

A depressed anterior fontanel is indicative of infant dehydration, which should be reported to the healthcare provider immediately. Rapid breathing and a weak, rapid pulse are other signs of infant dehydration.

A is incorrect because hyperactive bowel sounds are consistent with diarrhea and not a reason to contact the healthcare provider.

C is incorrect because 72 mL pale yellow urine is normal for an 8-month-old who weighs 18-lbs. Normal urine output for an infant is 1-3 ml/kg/hr. The converted weight is 8.16 kg, so the expected normal output for this child is 8-25 ml/hr. If the child's urinary output was less than 8 mL/hr., this would indicate dehydration.

D is incorrect because skin tenting is a sign of dehydration. If the nurse notes an absence of skin turgor, this indicates the patient is adequately hydrated and this does not need to be reported to the healthcare provider.

17. A 3-year-old girl is admitted to the pediatric medical-surgical unit with gastroenteritis. Which of the following interventions does the nurse initiate to prevent the spread of disease?

   A. Observe standard precautions
   B. Administer antibiotics as soon as possible
   C. Send a stool sample to the lab for culture
   D. Provide the patient with eating utensils which can be sterilized

Rationale:

Correct answer: A

Gastroenteritis is irritation and inflammation of the stomach and intestinal lining, which is usually viral and highly contagious. Standard precautions should be used when caring for the child with gastroenteritis.

B is incorrect because antibiotics are not generally used for treating gastroenteritis unless a specific bacterial agent has been identified as the cause. Treatment typically includes increased oral fluids, IV fluids if necessary to maintain hydration, and anti-parasitic drugs if the cause is a parasite.

C is incorrect because the purpose of sending a stool sample to the lab for culture is to determine the infection-causing agent, not to prevent the spread if the illness.

D is incorrect because eating utensils for a patient with gastroenteritis should be disposable.

18. The nurse is reviewing the medical record of a 3-week-old boy admitted for Hirschsprung's disease. Which of the following symptoms led the parents to seek care for the infant?

   A. Diaphragmatic pain
   B. Vomiting

C. Regurgitation
D. Foul smelling, ribbon-like stool

Rationale:

Correct answer: D

Hirschsprung's disease is a disease of the large intestine that interferes with the passage of stool due to nerve cells missing from the colon at birth. Inadequate motility causes mechanical obstruction of the intestine. Chronic constipation, due to the condition, causes foul smelling, ribbon-like stool.

A is incorrect because diaphragmatic pain is not common in Hirschsprung's disease, and a 3-week-old infant is not able to communicate such specific pain.

B is incorrect because vomiting is not a finding in Hirschsprung's disease.

C is incorrect because regurgitation is not a finding in Hirschsprung's disease.

19. The nurse is caring for a 3-month-old girl diagnosed with intussusception. When assessing the infant, which of the following does the nurse expect to find?

A. Watery diarrhea
B. Ribbon-like stool
C. Profuse, projectile vomiting
D. Blood and mucous in stools

Rationale:

Correct answer: D

Intussusception is invagination of the intestines into adjoining intestinal lumen which causes bowel obstruction. Symptoms include blood and mucous in stool, severe cramping and abdominal pain, and currant jelly-like stool.

A is incorrect because watery diarrhea is not characteristic of intussusception.

B is incorrect because ribbon-like stool is not characteristic of intussusception but rather a common finding with Hirschsprung's disease.

C is incorrect because profuse, projectile vomiting is not characteristic of intussusception.

20. The nurse is teaching the parents of a 2-year-old with a hernia about hernia strangulation signs. The nurse would inform the parents which sign would require notification of the healthcare provider?

    A. Fever
    B. Diarrhea
    C. Vomiting
    D. Foul-smelling stool

Rationale:

Correct answer: C

A hernia is protrusion of a section of the intestine through a weak spot in the abdominal wall. A strangulated hernia is a medical emergency in which the blood supply to the affected area of the intestine is cut off. The nurse would inform the parents of symptoms of a strangulated hernia: vomiting, severe abdominal pain, abdominal distention, and intestinal obstruction, any of which requires notification of the healthcare provider.

A is incorrect because fever may require notification of the healthcare provider but is not a sign of strangulation.

B is incorrect because diarrhea does not occur with a strangulated hernia.

D is incorrect because foul-smelling stool is not consistent with a strangulated hernia.

21. The nurse is teaching the parents of a child diagnosed with hepatitis A about care and prevention of transmission. Which of the following statements by the parents indicates more education is needed?

    A. "Handwashing is important."
    B. "We should feed our child a high-fat diet."
    C. "We will clean contaminated surfaces with bleach."
    D. "We understand that early treatment with gamma-globulins can help our child."

    Rationale:

    Correct answer: B

    Hepatitis is inflammation of the liver due to viral infection. In order to provide rest for the liver, a low-fat diet should be offered to the child.

    A is incorrect because handwashing is appropriate with hepatitis A as it is commonly transmitted on the hands after fecal contamination.

    C is incorrect because cleaning with bleach is appropriate in a home in which a person with hepatitis A is living.

    D is incorrect because it is a true statement; early treatment with gamma-globulin A post-exposure is beneficial to the patient with hepatitis A.

22. The nursing student on the pediatric medical unit is learning about phenylketonuria (PKU). The nursing student learns what about PKU?

    A. That it is an autosomal-dominant disorder

B. That it primarily affects the gastrointestinal system
C. Treatment includes restricting tyramine
D. All states require screening for the disorder

Rationale:

Correct answer: D

PKU is an autosomal recessive disorder of metabolism that causes buildup of phenylalanine in the body. Intellectual delay, seizures, behavioral problems, and mental disorders can result if PKU goes untreated. All states require infant screening for PKU.

A is incorrect because PKU is an autosomal recessive disorder, which means that both parents carry the gene, even though neither may show symptoms of the condition. In addition to PKU, cystic fibrosis, Tay-Sach's disease, and sickle cell disease are also autosomal recessive. Autosomal-dominant disorders require only one parent to pass the gene to the offspring. Marfan syndrome, Von Willebrand disease, and Huntington's disease are autosomal dominant.

B is incorrect because PKU affects all body systems.

C is incorrect because treatment of PKU includes restriction of phenylalanine, not tyramine.

23. The nurse in the pediatric emergency room is caring for an 18-month-old who has been experiencing vomiting. The nurse places the toddler in which position for sleep?

A. Supine
B. Side-lying
C. Prone with head elevated
D. Prone with head turned sideways

Rationale:

Correct answer: B

It is important to maintain the airway and prevent aspiration in a child who is vomiting. Side-lying is the most appropriate position to place the child.

A is incorrect because supine increases the risk of aspiration.

C is incorrect because prone with head elevated will not prevent aspiration.

D is incorrect because prone with head turned sideways will not prevent aspiration.

24. The nurse is caring for a 2-week-old infant and notes the healthcare provider has recorded a suspected diagnosis of esophageal atresia with tracheoesophageal fistula (TEF). Which of the following statements is appropriate for the nurse to make when discussing care with the infant's parents?

    A. "The initial TEF treatments are usually successful, and children with this anomaly rarely require surgery."
    B. "An oral feeding tube can provide your child with nutrition until the TEF has been corrected."
    C. "Choking with feeding is common with a TEF, so we will monitor closely for aspiration."
    D. "We will limit fluids through the child's peripheral IV to prevent fluid volume overload."

Rationale:

Correct answer: C

Tracheoesophageal fistula is a failure of the esophagus to develop as one continuous tube from the back of the pharynx down to the stomach. An opening can form between the esophagus and trachea, which is marked by coughing and choking during feeding and can cause cyanosis.

A is incorrect because TEF requires surgical repair.

B is incorrect because an oral feeding tube is not used in children with TEF. A gastrostomy tube or parenteral nutrition is used until the TEF is repaired surgically.

D is incorrect because babies with TEF generally receive fluids and antibiotics through an umbilical catheter, not a peripheral IV, and fluids need to be maintained, not limited.

25. The nurse in the neonatal intensive care unit (NICU) is caring for an infant diagnosed with pyloric stenosis. When assessing the infant, which of the following does the nurse expect to find?

   A. Watery diarrhea
   B. Projectile vomiting
   C. Increased urine output
   D. Vomiting large amounts of bile

Rationale:

Correct answer: B

Hypertrophic pyloric stenosis is obstruction of the gastric outlet due to hypertrophy and hyperplasia of the pylorus, which is the most common cause of vomiting in infants. Symptoms include projectile vomiting, irritability, hunger, crying, dehydration, decreased urine output, and constipation.

A is incorrect because constipation is associated with pyloric stenosis due to decreased stomach contents moving into the small intestine for absorption.

C is incorrect because decreased urine output is associated with pyloric stenosis due to dehydration from decreased water absorption.

D is incorrect because non-bilious vomiting is associated with pyloric stenosis.

CHAPTER 7:

NCLEX-RN – PEDIATRIC: INTEGUMENTARY - 25 QUESTIONS

1. The nurse in the pediatric emergency room is caring for a toddler who sustained burns on the upper torso from a house fire. Which of the following nursing diagnoses is highest priority for this child?

   A. Potential ineffective airway clearance related to edema of respiratory passages
   B. Impaired physical mobility related to disease process
   C. Disturbed sleep pattern related to facility environment
   D. Risk for infection related to impaired skin integrity

   Rationale:

   Correct answer: A

   Any time a child sustains burns to the upper torso, upper extremities, face, head, or neck, the primary goal of the nurse is to maintain integrity of the respiratory system. Airway clearance and reducing or preventing edema of respiratory passages are highest priorities in this scenario.

   B is incorrect because burns are not a disease, and physical mobility is not as concerning as airway clearance and effective air exchange.

C is incorrect because the patient is likely to have a disturbed sleep pattern which can impact healing, but this is not a greater priority than airway. The nurse and care team must carefully consider the plan of care to provide both stimulation and also time for adequate rest.

D is incorrect because risk for infection is a high priority but not more concerning than airway.

2. The nurse in the pediatric burn unit is caring for a toddler who sustained burns to both lower extremities due to scalding bath water. When caring for this child, which nursing intervention will assist with preventing contractures of the legs?

   A. Applying knee splints
   B. Elevating the foot of the bed
   C. Hyperextending the toddler's palms
   D. Performing shoulder range of motion exercises twice daily

Rationale:

Correct answer: A

Contractures are limitation of muscle and ligament motion due to burns, injury, or immobility. To prevent contractures, joints should be kept in a neutral position. Application of knee splints will hold the knees in a functional position and prevent contracture of the knee joints. Other nursing interventions to prevent contractures include applying shoes to prevent foot drop and providing range of motion (ROM) activities with each dressing change. The nurse determines whether to provide active or passive ROM based on the extent of tissue damage and the client's ability to move their own extremity.

B is incorrect because elevating the foot of the bed can help reduce edema but will not prevent contractures.

C is incorrect because hyperextending any joint for an extended time can cause contractures, and the palms are not at risk for contractures in a child who sustained burns to the lower extremities.

D is incorrect because shoulder range of motion exercises will not prevent contractures of the legs.

3. The parents of a 12-year-old girl bring her to the healthcare provider's office for a severe sunburn. When instructing the parents regarding adequate skin protection, which of the following is best for preventing future skin damage?

   A. "Minimize your child's sun exposure from 1 to 4 p.m., when the sun is at its strongest."
   B. "Use sunscreen with sun protection factor of 6 or more and cover all parts of the body."
   C. "Apply sunscreen regularly, even when the weather is overcast."
   D. "When you go to the beach, sit in the shade to prevent sunburn."

Rationale:

Correct answer: C

Sunscreen is most effective at preventing skin damage when it is used consistently, even when it is overcast.

A is incorrect because sun exposure should be minimized between 10 am and 2 pm, when the sun is strongest.

B is incorrect because SPF 15 or greater should be recommended and should be applied to all skin that is potentially going to be exposed to the sun.

D is incorrect because sitting in shade while at the beach is not as effective at preventing sunburn as regularly using SPF of 15 or greater.

4. A 13-year-old boy is in the dermatology clinic with his parents for psoriasis. When assessing the affected areas, which of the following types of secondary lesions does the nurse expect to find?

   A. Scale
   B. Crust
   C. Ulcer
   D. Scar

Rationale:

Correct answer: A

Psoriasis is caused by an autoimmune disease that leads to red, raised, thick, itchy plaques on the skin covered by silvery-white scales with symmetrical distribution. These lesions are most commonly found on the elbows, knees, scalp, sacrum, and behind the ears. Scales are secondary lesions in psoriasis.

B is incorrect because crust is not found with psoriasis.

C is incorrect because ulcers are not found with psoriasis.

D is incorrect because scars may be present on the skin from previous outbreaks but are not a secondary lesion found with psoriasis.

5. The nurse is planning to administer dexamethasone topical cream to a school-age child with dermatitis on the anterior chest. How does the nurse apply the topical agent?

   A. Using a circular motion to enhance absorption
   B. Upward motion to increase blood supply to the affected area
   C. Long, even, outward, and downward strokes
   D. After washing the affected area with soap and warm water

Rationale:

Correct answer: C

In a child with eczematous dermatitis (or atopic dermatitis), the nurse will note rough, dry, erythematous skin lesions that progress to weeping and crusting. Skin may appear blistered and swollen. Topical steroids and antihistamine agents should be applied beginning at the midline and using long, even, outward, and downward strokes to reduce follicle irritation and skin inflammation. The client's fingernails should be kept short and clean, and non-irritating loose cotton clothing should be worn to minimize itching and discomfort.

A is incorrect because using a circular motion can cause follicle irritation and skin inflammation.

B is incorrect because upward motion can cause follicle irritation and skin inflammation.

D is incorrect because soap can be irritating to the skin in a patient with eczema. A warm colloid bath solution is best for cleansing the skin, if necessary.

6. A 9-year-old girl is admitted to the emergency room for frostbite to the toes after playing in the snow for several hours. When assessing the girl, which of the following characteristics would the nurse expect to find?

   A. Gangrenous, edematous toes
   B. Bright red skin and nail beds edematous
   C. Slurred speech
   D. White skin insensitive to touch

Rationale:

Correct answer: D

Frostbite occurs when skin and possibly underlying tissues are exposed to cold temperatures for a prolonged period of time. Skin that is frostbitten is white or blue in color, and the skin is cold, hard, and insensitive to touch. Frostbite is common on the ears, nose, cheeks, chin, fingers, and toes.

A is incorrect because edema is characteristic of frostbite, but gangrene is a late complication which does not appear after several hours of cold exposure.

B is incorrect because bright red skin and edematous nailbeds are not characteristic of frostbite.

C is incorrect because slurred speech is characteristic of hypothermia, not specifically frostbite.

7. The nurse is caring for four patients on the pediatric medical unit. Which patient needs to be evaluated for wound infection?

   A. Patient with a uniform bed of granulation tissue across the wound
   B. Patient whose wound has thin, serous drainage
   C. Patient whose white blood cell count was 24,000/mm^3 this morning
   D. Patient whose wound is decreasing in size

Rationale:

Correct answer: C

Normal white blood cell (WBC) count is 4,500-10,000/mm^3. An elevated WBC count indicates possible infection, so this patient should be assessed for wound infection. Other indications of wound infection include viscous/purulent drainage, discoloration of tissue within the wound and at the wound margins, or unexpected pain during dressing change or when the dressing is in place.

A is incorrect because a uniform bed of granulation tissue suggests the wound is healing properly. An indication of wound infection is strips of granulation tissue at the base of the wound.

B is incorrect because thin, serous drainage from a wound is not an indication of wound infection.

D is incorrect because a wound decreasing in size is not an indication of wound infection.

8. A 16-year-old boy in the clinic has multiple lesions of the skin. Which of the following lesions should be evaluated by the nurse first?

   A. Beige freckles on the hands and arms
   B. Lower leg mole, irregular shape, blue with white specks
   C. Cluster of pustules to the left axilla
   D. Red, thick pustules with white scales on the chest

Rationale:

Correct answer: B

A mole that is irregular and blue with white specks fits criteria for possibly being precancerous or cancerous and must be investigated immediately. The criteria for cancer include variation of color in one lesion, irregular border, size greater than 6mm, and change in appearance or new symptom.

A is incorrect because freckles are benign.

C is incorrect because pustules indicate possible infection, but a potential cancerous lesion should be assessed first.

D is incorrect because red, thick pustules with white scales describe psoriasis, which is chronic and autoimmune, and not the nurse's greatest priority.

9. The nurse is documenting a wound assessment for a 7-year-old boy who was injured in a motor vehicle accident. The nurse notes the presence of a scab on a deep wound. Which phase of wound healing does the nurse identify this as?

   A. Inflammatory
   B. Migratory
   C. Proliferative
   D. Maturation

Rationale:

Correct answer: B

Wound healing progresses through several stages including inflammation, proliferation, migration, and reepithelialization. Scab formation occurs in the migratory phase due to epithelial cell migration, fibroblast synthesis of scar tissue, and new cells developing across a wound.

A is incorrect because during the inflammatory stage, the scab has not yet formed. The inflammatory stage is marked by redness and swelling while damaged and dead cells are cleared out, along with bacteria and other pathogens or debris. White blood cells engulf debris within the wound by the process of phagocytosis during the inflammatory stage.

C is incorrect because the scab has not yet formed in the proliferative stage. This stage of wound healing is characterized by granulation tissue filling the wound and contraction of the wound edges.

D is incorrect because the maturation phase is sloughing off of the scab and return of the skin to normal.

10. The nurse in the pediatric unit is caring for a toddler with severe impetigo. Which of the following interventions does the nurse include in the child's plan of care?

    A. Placing mitts on the child's hands
    B. Administering systemic antibiotics
    C. Applying topical antibiotics
    D. Continuing to administer antibiotics for 21 days as prescribed

Rationale:

Correct answer: B

Impetigo is a superficial skin infection due to beta-hemolytic streptococci or staphylococci and is contagious. Severe impetigo requires 7 to 10 days of systemic antibiotics to prevent glomerulonephritis.

A is incorrect because the toddler's nails should be trimmed to prevent scratching. Mitts are used for infants with impetigo to prevent secondary infection, but mitts should be avoided with toddlers because they are a form of restraint, and the toddler can follow directions and be discouraged from scratching.

C is incorrect because topical antibiotics are not as effective for severe impetigo.

D is incorrect because antibiotics are administered for 7 to 10 days.

11. The nurse in the pediatric emergency room admits a 10-year-old boy with external bleeding from the right lower extremity. What is the nurse's initial intervention?

    A. Elevation of the extremity
    B. Pressure point control
    C. Application of direct pressure
    D. Application of a tourniquet

Rationale:

Correct answer: C

Direct pressure application is the first step in controlling external bleeding. Placing direct pressure on the wound restricts blood flow manually. The nurse should use a sterile barrier (such as gauze) to help reduce the risk for infection while applying direct pressure to the point of bleeding.

A is incorrect because elevation reduces flow to the affected extremity and can decrease bleeding, but direct pressure must be applied to the site of hemorrhage before elevation.

B is incorrect because pressure point control is used only after direct pressure and elevation fail to control the bleeding. Pressure point control involves constricting the major artery that feeds the point of the bleed. A major risk of using the pressure point method is necrosis below the point of constriction.

D is incorrect because a tourniquet (band tied tightly around the limb to restrict blood flow) is only used to decrease bleeding if all other measures have failed. Often times, a tourniquet can fail to stop bleeding and even increase bleeding by impairing venous blood flow.

12. The father of a 7-year-old boy calls the clinic nurse to report that his son has come into contact with poison ivy. When the father asks the nurse if there is a treatment that can prevent the poison ivy rash from occurring, what is the first question the nurse should ask?

    A. “Have you had your son take a shower?”
    B. “Does your son have any sign of a rash yet?”
    C. “Do you have any oral or topical antihistamines on hand?”
    D. “Is your son allergic to poison ivy?”

Rationale:

Correct answer: A

When poison ivy sap comes into contact with skin, it's oil, urushiol, forms an invisible film on skin. Up to 85 percent of Americans will develop an allergic contact dermatitis rash when directly in contact with this oil. Showering with copious lathering and rinsing is the first intervention after coming in contact with poison ivy, so this is the first question that should be asked.

B is incorrect because the rash from poison ivy does not occur immediately after contact. Itchy blisters or a streaky red rash may occur within hours up to 2 days after contact, and usually last 1 to 2 weeks. The blisters may weep and eventually crust over.

C is incorrect because antihistamines are not used until after the skin has been thoroughly washed and all clothing which may have come into contact with the poison ivy has been changed.

D is incorrect because it is an inappropriate question for the nurse to ask and will not necessarily be helpful at this time. Not all individuals are allergic to the oil (urushiol) from a poison ivy plant, but people rarely know if they are allergic or not (roughly 75 to 85 percent of people are allergic).

13. The community health nurse has provided education regarding prevention of Lyme disease. Which statement by a child indicates more teaching is needed?

    A. "We shouldn't use insect repellants because they attract ticks."
    B. "Wearing long-sleeved tops and pants is important."
    C. "We should wear hats when we go hiking."
    D. "We should wear closed-toed shoes and socks that can be pulled up over our pants."

Rationale:

Correct answer: A

Lyme disease is a bacterial disease caused by *Borrelia burgdorferi* and transmitted to humans from infected ticks. The best way to prevent Lyme disease is to avoid wooded areas with tall grass. Prevention of Lyme disease also includes wearing insect repellant (20% DEET or higher is recommended), wearing long-sleeved tops and pants, wearing hats, and closed-toed shoes and long socks pulled over the pants. Gloves may also be worn, tucked into the sleeves of the shirt to prevent ticks from crawling up the wrists.

B is incorrect because wearing long-sleeved tops and pants will help prevent Lyme disease. Clothing should be changed after spending time outdoors, as ticks may remain on clothing for several hours before attaching to the skin.

C is incorrect because wearing hats will help prevent ticks from hiding in the hair and potentially attaching to the scalp.

D is incorrect because wearing closed-toed shoes and long socks will prevent Lyme disease.

14. The student nurse in the pediatric intensive care unit (ICU) is learning about monitoring for cyanosis in dark-skinned children. The student learns that the area least optimal to assess for cyanosis is:

   A. Nail beds
   B. Lips
   C. Sclera of the eye
   D. Tongue

Rationale:

Correct answer: C

Cyanosis occurs when an increased amount of unoxygenated blood circulates. Cyanosis reflects compromised oxygen saturation and causes a blue-gray or whitish tinge to the lips, tongue, oral mucosa, nail beds, conjunctivae, and palms and soles of the hands and feet in dark-skinned children. The nurse may also observe for cyanotic skin color changes over the cheekbones and on the earlobes. The sclera is not optimal for assessing for cyanosis in dark-skinned children. (Note: other indications of decreased tissue perfusion include cold, clammy skin, a rapid, thread pulse, and rapid, shallow respirations.)

A is incorrect because nail beds are appropriate to assess for cyanosis.

B is incorrect because lips are appropriate to assess for cyanosis.

D is incorrect because the tongue is appropriate to assess for cyanosis.

15. The nurse in the pediatric clinic is assessing a 4-year-old child with folliculitis. Which of the following assessment findings does the nurse expect?

    A. Bullous formations on the skin
    B. Deep localized infection
    C. Numbness at the infection site
    D. Reddened, raised hair follicles

Rationale:

Correct answer: D

Folliculitis is inflammation of hair follicles due to infection of either bacterial or fungal origin. It appears as reddened, raised hair follicles. Lesions may be superficial or deep. Single or multiple papules or pustules may appear within or close to the hair follicles. Folliculitis most commonly appears within a man's beard, or on the legs of ladies who shave. Other areas include the axillae, trunk, or buttocks.

A is incorrect because bullous formations (large, fluid-filled vesicles) on the skin is characteristic of impetigo, often caused by *S. aureus*. The face, hands, and neck are most commonly involved, and the bullae can rupture, leaving raw, reddened areas. Impetigo is highly contagious.

B is incorrect because deep localized infection is characteristic of cellulitis. Skin will appear swollen, red, hot, and tender, and often pits when pressed by the fingertips. When cellulitis affects deep tissues under the skin, it can become a systemic, life-threatening infection.

C is incorrect because folliculitis is characterized by itching and soreness at the infection site.

16. A 9-year-old girl is in the family practice clinic with impetigo. When instructing the parents on how to care for the skin infection, which of the following does the nurse recommend?

    A. Squeezing of vesicles
    B. Antibiotics
    C. Soaking in an ice bath
    D. Placing gloves on the child to prevent scratching

Rationale:

Correct answer: B

Impetigo is a superficial skin infection due to beta-hemolytic streptococci and is contagious. Crusts must be gently removed from vesicles in order for topical antibiotics (polysporin or bacitracin) to work to clear the infection. Topical antibiotics are generally used for treating impetigo when it is limited to a small area; however, systemic antibiotics may be needed if reduce the contagious spread and treat deep infection.

A is incorrect because squeezing of vesicles is not recommended as this can increase the spread of impetigo and cause unnecessary pain.

C is incorrect because soaking in an ice bath is not recommended. The nurse should teach the patient with impetigo to wash the lesions with a warm soap solution or to use povidone-iodine or chlorhexidine to remove the crust and effect the central site of bacterial growth.

D is incorrect because placing gloves on the child is not necessary. As impetigo is highly contagious, the infected child should avoid contact with other children or individuals at risk for infection until 24 hours after the antibiotic therapy has begun. The parent or healthcare provider should wear gloves when caring for the lesions of a child with impetigo.

17. The parents of a 6-month-old have brought the infant to the pediatric clinic for diaper rash. Which of the following suggestions does the nurse make to assist with improving the diaper rash?

    A. Change diapers less often
    B. Apply steroid cream
    C. Apply talc
    D. Apply skin barrier cream

Rationale:

Correct answer: D

Diaper rash is inflammation and irritation of the skin in the perineal or groin area due to constant exposure to wetness. Skin contact with urine or feces containing urea, enzymes, and bacteria combined with a baby's sensitive skin can contribute to diaper rash. Other causative factors include the beginning of the introduction of solid foods to infants, diapers and clothes that are too tight, and the use of antibiotics. More frequent diaper changes, exposing the area to air, skin barrier cream, and cornstarch are all recommended treatments for diaper rash.

A is incorrect because diapers should be changed more often, every 2 to 3 hours to prevent diaper rash.

B is incorrect because steroid creams are not recommended to treat diaper rash unless specifically prescribed by the healthcare provider.

C is incorrect because talc is not recommended. Parents should also be encouraged to use a soft cloth moistened with water, instead of prepackaged wet wipes, as these wipes may contain chemicals that are irritating to the skin and can worsen diaper rash.

18. The nurse in the pediatric clinic is caring for a 6-year-old boy with tinea corporis. Which of the following interventions does the nurse perform for this condition?

    A. Systemic antibiotics
    B. Skin scrub with betadine
    C. Topical therapy
    D. Radiotherapy

Rationale:

Correct answer: C

Tinea corporis is a fungal infection of the skin (ringworm of the body, not on the feet or scalp). This superficial condition is characterized by annular, raised rings on the skin. Tinea corporis is typically treated with topical therapy with -azole drugs or allylamines. Affected areas should be washed frequently and kept clean and dry. Other types of tinea include tinea pedis (athlete's foot) and tinea capitis (ringworm on the scalp).

A is incorrect because systemic antibiotics are not usually used, as ringworm is caused by a fungus. Antibiotics will only be needed if the initial infection causes a secondary bacterial, more extensive infection.

B is incorrect because betadine scrub is not indicated for tinea corporis.

D is incorrect because radiotherapy is not indicated for tinea corporis. Radiotherapy (teletherapy) can be internal or external radiation treatment used for some cancers, not fungal infections.

19. A nurse is preparing to see a 4-year-old child in the pediatric unit with atopic dermatitis. Which of the following manifestations does the nurse expect to find?

    A. Inflamed, red, swollen, itchy skin
    B. Annular, raised rings
    C. Pustules
    D. Smooth, red skin

Rationale:

Correct answer: A

Atopic dermatitis (eczema) is a red rash that evolves rapidly and is blistered and swollen. It appears as inflamed, red, swollen, and itchy skin. The skin lesions may progress to weeping and crusting. Parents should be taught to eliminate offending foods in the child's diet which may cause the eczema, such as milk, eggs, wheat, citrus fruits, or tomatoes. Irritating clothing (rough fabric or wool) that promotes sweating can also trigger eczema in children. Cotton clothing is best. Soap and long or hot baths and showers should be avoided. Topical steroids and antihistamines may be used to treat eczema.

B is incorrect because annular, raised rings are characteristic of tinea corporis, ringworm fungal infection of skin on the body (not the scalp or feet).

C is incorrect because pustules are not characteristic of eczema. Pustules are commonly seen with folliculitis, impetigo, or acne vulgaris.

D is incorrect because skin affected by eczema is rough and dry.

20. The parents of a 6-year-old boy diagnosed with eczema ask the nurse how the skin condition occurs. What is the best response by the nurse?

A. "Eczema is caused by irritants such as poison ivy."
B. "Eczema is caused by a trigger antigen and the inflammatory process."
C. "It is a genetic condition."
D. "It is caused by varicella."

Rationale:

Correct answer: B

Atopic dermatitis or eczema is a red rash that evolves rapidly and is blistered and swollen. Eczema is started by a trigger antigen which leads to the inflammatory process, rash, and itching due to the rash. The trigger antigen may be a certain food in the diet (commonly milk, eggs, wheat, citrus fruits, or tomatoes) or by tight, irritating clothing such as wool, which can promote sweating.

A is incorrect because poison ivy causes allergic eczema, not atopic dermatitis.

C is incorrect because eczema may be a precursor to adult asthma or hay fever but is not genetic.

D is incorrect because varicella does not cause eczema.

21. The nurse is preparing to admit a 9-year-old boy with varicella-zoster. What type of isolation precautions does the nurse implement?

A. Positive pressure isolation room
B. Only standard precautions
C. Airborne precautions
D. Droplet precautions

Rationale:

Correct answer: C.

Varicella-zoster, or chicken pox, is an infection of the skin caused by the varicella-zoster virus. The nurse should implement airborne and contact precautions as varicella-zoster is spread through coughing, sneezing, and saliva, as well as contact with blisters or contaminated objects. Prodromal signs include a slight fever, malaise, and decreased appetite. The rash associated with varicella-zoster is pruritic and begins as macule, then progresses to a papule, and then a vesicle. Successive crops of all three stages may be present at any one time. Other findings include lymphadenopathy and elevated temperature.

A is incorrect because varicella-zoster requires airborne precautions until the lesions are crusted over. Airborne precautions involve the use of a negative-pressure isolation room, in which contaminated air from the patient's room is removed via a pressurized system that does not allow that air to circulate back through the hospital's ventilatory system.

B is incorrect because standard precautions are not enough when caring for a patient with varicella-zoster.

D is incorrect because varicella-zoster is not spread by droplet transmission.

22. A father calls the pediatric clinic to speak with the nurse about his 5-year-old daughter who has cold symptoms, fever, and red bumps all over the body. Which of the following does the nurse suspect?

  A. Eczema
  B. Impetigo
  C. Tinea corporis
  D. Varicella-zoster

Rationale:

Correct answer: D

Varicella-zoster, or chicken pox, is an infection of the skin caused by the varicella-zoster virus. It is characterized by cold symptoms, fever, and red bumps all over the body.

A is incorrect because eczema is generally found on the cheeks, scalp, in elbow joints, and behind the knees, not all over the body.

B is incorrect because impetigo is characterized by reddish-colored macules which turn into honey-colored crusted vesicles.

C is incorrect because tinea corporis, a fungal infection, is characterized by annular, raised rings on the skin.

23. The nursing student is learning about acne vulgaris. The student learns which ages are most often affected by acne vulgaris?

    A. 15-18 years
    B. 1-3 years
    C. 4-6 years
    D. 7-10 years

Rationale:

Correct answer: A

Acne vulgaris is blockage and inflammation of hair follicles and sebaceous glands, most commonly affecting the skin on the face, back, neck, and chest. Blackheads, whiteheads, papules, pustules, and cysts are common. Children most affected by acne vulgaris ae ages 15 to 18 years. Treatment includes PO tetracycline and other antibiotic agents. Nursing considerations include providing emotional support and monitoring for secondary infection.

B is incorrect because 1 to 3-year-old children do not commonly get acne vulgaris.

C is incorrect because 4 to 6-year-olds do not get acne vulgaris.

D is incorrect because 7 to 10-year-olds can begin to develop acne vulgaris but are not most often affected by it.

24. A 16-year-old boy is in the family practice clinic for acne vulgaris. When the boy asks the nurse the best way to deal with the acne, what does the nurse recommend?

    A. Squeeze the pustules
    B. Wash the skin with hot water
    C. Alcohol rinse
    D. Benzoyl peroxide

Rationale:

Correct answer: D

Acne vulgaris is blockage and inflammation of hair follicles and sebaceous glands affecting the face, back, neck, and chest. Treatment includes benzoyl peroxide, typically applied to the affected areas in gel, cream, or liquid, in concentrations of 2.5% increasing through 5.0%, and up to 10%. Other medications may include tetracycline antibiotics, retinoid-like agents, and hormones. Nursing priorities include teaching the adolescent about good nutrition and hygiene and providing emotional support.

A is incorrect because squeezing acne pustules can worsen acne, prolong healing and cause unnecessary pain.

B is incorrect because hot water can worsen acne.

C is incorrect because alcohol is irritating to the skin and can worsen acne.

25. The nurse in the family practice clinic is caring for a 14-year-old with acne vulgaris who is concerned about his appearance. Which of the following nursing diagnoses does the nurse implement for this patient?

   A. Activity intolerance related to acne vulgaris
   B. Disturbed body image related to acne vulgaris
   C. Skin infection related to acne vulgaris
   D. Deficient knowledge related to acne vulgaris

Rationale:

Correct answer: B

Acne vulgaris is blockage and inflammation of hair follicles and sebaceous glands affecting the face, back, and chest. This can cause psychological distress due to the appearance of pustules and redness of the skin. Disturbed body image is the most appropriate nursing diagnosis for this adolescent related to his concern about his appearance.

A is incorrect because activity intolerance is not common in adolescents experiencing acne.

C is incorrect because skin infection is not a nursing diagnosis.

D is incorrect because the adolescent is expressing concern about his image, not a lack of knowledge about acne or its treatment plan.

CHAPTER 8:

NCLEX-RN – PEDIATRIC: ONCOLOGY & GENETICS - 25 QUESTIONS

1. A 9-year-old boy diagnosed with leukemia has completed his first treatment with chemotherapy. When providing discharge instructions to the parents, which of the following does the nurse include?

    A. Provide a low-protein, high-carbohydrate diet
    B. Avoid fresh vegetables that are not peeled or cooked
    C. Notify the healthcare provider if his temperature is greater than 101°F (39°C)
    D. Increase use of humidifiers in the house

Rationale:

Correct answer: B

Leukemia is a malignant neoplastic disease which causes increased numbers of abnormal or immature leukocytes to be produced from the bone marrow and blood-forming organs, suppressing normal blood cell production. The patient is at increased risk for infection. Vegetables and fruits can harbor microorganisms which can lead to infections in the immunocompromised child. All fruits and vegetables should be peeled or cooked.

A is incorrect because a low-protein diet is not indicated in leukemia. A low-protein diet may be necessary for a patient with renal disease or phenylketonuria.

C is incorrect because leukemia patients may have an infectious process in the body without a significant rise in temperature. Thus, the healthcare provider should be notified for temperature greater than 100°F.

D is incorrect because humidifiers can harbor microorganisms and fungi, increasing the risk for infection in the home. The leukemia patient does not need increased humidity in the air.

2. A 6-year-old girl diagnosed with hemophilia type A is in the emergency room after falling off her bicycle. The nurse assesses the child and finds the knee is extensively swollen. What is the first action the nurse should perform?

    A. Initiate a peripheral IV to administer cryoprecipitate
    B. Type and crossmatch for transfusion
    C. Monitor the child's vital signs for the first five minutes
    D. Apply an ice pack and compression dressing to the knee

Rationale:

Correct answer: D

Hemophilia type A is a hereditary lack of coagulation factors which severely reduces the clotting ability of the blood. Rest, ice, compression, and elevation (RICE) should be initiated immediately to reduce swelling and bleeding into the knee, which is priority in hemophilia.

A is incorrect because prior to administering cryoprecipitate, the nurse must apply ice to the site of the injury.

B is incorrect because type and crossmatch is not a priority until after ice is applied to reduce blood flow to the area of injury.

C is incorrect because vital signs may not indicate early bleeding. The nursing priority is to reduce the likelihood of bleeding.

3. A husband and wife both have the sickle cell trait and ask the nurse about the possibility of their children inheriting sickle cell disease. What is the most appropriate response by the nurse?

   A. One child will have sickle cell disease
   B. Only male children will be affected
   C. Each pregnancy carries a 25 percent chance of the child being affected
   D. If four children are born, one will have sickle cell disease

Rationale:

Correct answer: C

Sickle cell disease is a hereditary anemia which mutates hemoglobin and distorts red blood cells to a sickle or crescent shape when oxygen levels are low. It is an autosomal recessive trait, and with both parents being carriers, there is a 25 percent chance each of their children will have sickle cell disease.

A is incorrect because there is a 25 percent chance each child will have sickle cell disease. The nurse cannot make a definitive prognosis of a single child having the disease.

B is incorrect because the disease can affect both male and female children.

D is incorrect because there is a 25 percent chance each child will have sickle cell disease, but this is not a guarantee that one of four children will definitively develop the disease.

4. The nurse is teaching the parents of a 6-year-old girl with sickle cell disease. When addressing sickle cell crisis, which of the following should the nurse include?

   A. Sickle cell crisis results from altered metabolism and dehydration
   B. Primary problems are due to tissue hypoxia and vascular occlusion
   C. Increased bilirubin levels lead to hypertension
   D. Clotting factors decrease with increased white blood cells

Rationale:

Correct answer: B

Sickle cell disease is a hereditary anemia which mutates hemoglobin and distorts red blood cells to a sickle or crescent shape when oxygen levels are low. The oxygen-carrying capacity of red blood cells is decreased, leading to tissue hypoxia. Sickled cells clump together, leading to vascular occlusion.

A is incorrect because sickle cell crisis results from tissue hypoxia and vascular occlusion. (Dehydration should, however, be avoided in crisis because it can prolong or worsen the crisis.)

C is incorrect because bilirubin levels are not related to sickle cell crisis.

D is incorrect because clotting factors are not part of sickle cell crisis.

5. The nurse is interviewing the parents of a 3-year-old boy with Down syndrome. Which of the following goals of care does the nurse identify as appropriate for this child?

   A. Encourage self-care skills
   B. Teach the child something new each day
   C. Encourage lenient behavior limits
   D. Achieve age-appropriate social skills

Rationale:

Correct answer: A

Down syndrome is a genetic defect characterized by an extra chromosome, number 21. Common features include short stature, decreased muscle tone, large forehead, flattened facial features, low-set ears, a low nasal bridge, congenital heart defects, and intellectual disability. The IQ generally ranges from 20 to 70. The primary goal for Down syndrome is teaching independence and self-care as much as possible to promote optimal functioning.

B is incorrect because learning new things daily may not be possible for a child with Down syndrome.

C is incorrect because behavior standards and discipline should be consistent for a child with Down syndrome. Lenient behavior limits may lead to behavioral problems and inability to follow rules and learn to adapt to societal expectations.

D is incorrect because this is an unrealistic expectation: the child with Down syndrome may not be able to attain age-appropriate social skills.

6. The nurse is teaching the parents of a 2-year-old boy diagnosed with Duchenne's muscular dystrophy about the disease and management. Which statement by the parents indicates the teaching was successful?

   A. "My son will probably not be able to walk by the time he is 9 years old."
   B. "Muscle relaxants work for some children; I hope they help my son."
   C. "When my son is a little older, surgery can improve his ability to walk."
   D. "I must help my son be active as possible to prevent disease progression."

Rationale:

Correct answer: A

Muscular dystrophy is an X-linked recessive disorder transmitted by female carriers to affected sons 50 percent of the time. The disease is characterized by progressive muscle weakness, joint contractures, and lordosis/scoliosis. Children with this disease usually are unable to walk independently by the age of 9 years.

B is incorrect because muscle relaxants are not used to treat muscular dystrophy.

C is incorrect because there is no surgical treatment for muscular dystrophy. Treatment generally includes intensive physical therapy, active and passive range of motion exercises, and in best cases, long-leg braces to help with ambulation.

D is incorrect because no effective treatment has been found to delay the progression of muscular dystrophy. Muscular dystrophy is generally progressive and fatal.

7. A new mother has just been informed her newborn has Down syndrome. The nurse is preparing to assess the newborn at the beginning of the shift. Which characteristic does the nurse not associate with Down syndrome?

   A. Simian crease
   B. Brachycephaly
   C. Oily skin
   D. Hypotonicity

Rationale:

Correct answer: C

Down syndrome is a genetic defect that causes decreased muscle tone, large forehead, flattened facial features, congenital heart defects, and intellectual disability. Characteristics include Simian crease, brachycephaly, dry skin, and hypotonicity.

A is incorrect because Simian crease (also known as a single palmar crease) is associated with Down syndrome. Most people have three palmar creases, which develop while in utero. A single palmar crease is seen in people whose fetal development was interrupted, such as Down syndrome, Trisomy 13, and Fetal Alcohol Syndrome.

B is incorrect because brachycephaly is a shortened skull shape, associated with Down syndrome.

D is incorrect because hypotonicity (abnormally low muscle tone) is associated with Down syndrome.

8. The nurse in the pediatric unit is caring for a 6-year-old girl with cystic fibrosis. Which of the following is not part of the cystic fibrosis triad?

   A. Pancreatic enzyme deficiency
   B. Fever
   C. High concentration of sweat electrolytes
   D. COPD

Rationale:

Correct answer: B

Cystic fibrosis is a genetic disorder that affects exocrine production of mucous and sweat, causing dysfunction in the lungs and digestive system. The cystic fibrosis triad is pancreatic enzyme deficiency, high concentration of sweat electrolytes, and COPD. Fever is not part of the triad. However, fever in a cystic fibrosis patient may indication a lung infection, which increases the need for calories and protein.

A is incorrect because pancreatic enzyme deficiency is part of the cystic fibrosis triad. The patient often suffers from malabsorption of fat and fat-soluble vitamins and weight loss. Supplemental pancreatic enzymes are needed for lifelong replacement.

C is incorrect because high concentration of sweat electrolytes is part of the cystic fibrosis triad. Thickened secretions in the body include sweat and oral mucous.

D is incorrect because COPD is part of the cystic fibrosis triad and lung disease is common. Many cystic fibrosis patients require a lung transplant by the age of 25.

9. A child with cystic fibrosis is in the clinic with her mother reporting a cough and runny nose. The nurse teaches the child's mother to do which of the following?

   A. Make sure the child has adequate nutritional intake
   B. Take the child's temperature twice per day
   C. Offer plenty of orange juice
   D. Increase chest physiotherapy to four times daily

Rationale:

Correct answer: D

Cystic fibrosis is a genetic disorder that affects production of mucous and sweat, causing dysfunction in the lungs and digestive system. The child is displaying early signs of an upper respiratory tract infection, which can quickly develop into pneumonia for a child with cystic fibrosis. Pulmonary secretions must be loosened and removed with percussion and postural drainage.

A is incorrect because eating well is important in general for a child with cystic fibrosis. The child generally needs a low-fat, high-protein, high-calorie diet. However, with signs of a respiratory infection present, chest physiotherapy is a bigger priority than dietary needs.

B is incorrect because frequent assessment of the child's temperature is important but not as much as chest physiotherapy.

C is incorrect because a child with cystic fibrosis needs adequate hydration, and orange juice is not contraindicated, but chest physiotherapy is the greater priority. Foods to avoid with cystic fibrosis include peanut butter, milk, and other thick products or food items that can cause thickening of saliva.

10. The nurse in the pediatric medical-surgical unit is caring for a 10-year-old girl with cystic fibrosis. The child tells the nurse she feels like she isn't getting enough air. Which of the following assessments is of greatest concern to the nurse?

    A. Sunken abdomen
    B. Distended jugular veins
    C. Edema in upper extremities
    D. Clubbing of fingers and toes

Rationale:

Correct answer: D.

Cystic fibrosis is a genetic disorder that affects production of mucous and sweat, causing dysfunction in the lungs and digestive system. Clubbing of fingers and toes indicates collateral circulation has been built to compensate for decreased oxygen levels.

A is incorrect because a sunken abdomen is a sign of poor nutritional intake but not as concerning as respiratory decompensation.

B is incorrect because distended jugular veins can be a sign of fluid volume overload or superior vena cava syndrome but are not related to the patient's complaints that she is not getting enough air. The nurse's greatest concern is respiratory decompensation and hypoxia.

C is incorrect because edema in upper extremities is unrelated to decreased oxygen levels.

11. The mother of a 6-year-old patient with hemophilia type A has received instructions from the clinic nurse. Which of the following statements indicates a need for further education?

    A. "I understand my child should avoid taking ibuprofen because this medication can affect clotting factors."
    B. "We will encourage non-contact activities, such as swimming or golf."
    C. "Aspirin is contraindicated because of my child's age and diagnosis."
    D. "I understand that the treatment for hemophilia does not increase my child's risks for contracting diseases such as HIV and hepatitis C."

Rationale:

Correct answer: D

Hemophilia type A is a hereditary lack of coagulation factors which severely reduces the clotting ability of the blood. Treatment includes IV infusion of cryoprecipitate and factor VIII clotting factor, which are derived from blood products. Any time a patient receives blood products by transfusion, the risk for communicable diseases such as HIV and hepatitis C is increased.

A is incorrect because the statement indicates an understanding that ibuprofen affects clotting factors.

B is incorrect because it indicates an understanding that contact sports should be avoided due to the risk of easy bruising and bleeding with hemophilia.

C is incorrect because it indicates understanding that aspirin should be avoided in children and patients with hemophilia.

12. A 4-year-old boy is admitted to the pediatric oncology ward with a diagnosis of acute leukemia. Which of the following assessments is most concerning to the nurse?

    A. Abdominal pain and anorexia
    B. Fatigue and bruising
    C. Bleeding gums and pallor
    D. Weakness, weight loss, and mucosal ulcers

Rationale:

Correct answer: C

Acute leukemia is a malignant disease which causes increased numbers of abnormal or immature leukocytes to be produced from the bone marrow and blood-forming organs, suppressing normal blood cell production. Onset is generally quick and can progress to fatal termination within days to months. The child's leukocyte count will be elevated and platelet count will be low, so monitoring for bleeding and pallor is most important.

A is incorrect because abdominal pain and anorexia are common and expected findings with acute leukemia.

B is incorrect because fatigue and bruising are common findings in a child with leukemia and not as alarming as bleeding and pallor.

D is incorrect because weakness, weight loss, and mucosal ulcers are not signs of a life-threatening complication with acute leukemia.

13. A 2-year-old boy has been diagnosed with cystic fibrosis. The mother asks the nurse what the major concern is now and what will happen in the future. What is the best response by the nurse?

    A. "There is a probability of lifelong complications."
    B. "Cystic fibrosis results in nutritional concerns that can be dealt with."
    C. "Thin, tenacious secretions from the lungs are a constant struggle with cystic fibrosis."
    D. "You will have a team of experts and a support group you can attend."

Rationale:

Correct answer: C

Cystic fibrosis is a genetic disorder that affects production of mucous and sweat, causing dysfunction in the lungs and digestive system. The tenacious secretions from the lungs are a struggle to deal with in cystic fibrosis, so respiratory threats are of major concern. This is the best of the answer choices because this nursing response addresses the mother's question and gives information specific to the diagnosis.

A is incorrect because although it is a true statement, it is too vague. The nurse should give specific information related to the diagnosis and address the mother's question.

B is incorrect because although it is a true statement, nutritional concerns are not the highest concern. The nurse must give truthful information related to the diagnosis and include teaching about the greatest concern, which is the child's respiratory system.

D is incorrect because giving information about medical experts and support groups does not address the mother's question.

14. An 8-year-old girl is diagnosed with non-Hodgkin's lymphoma. The nurse knows the most urgent complication that must be evaluated at diagnosis and followed closely is which of the following?

    A. Elevated white blood cell count greater than 50,000/mm^3
    B. Uric acid 5.0
    C. Mediastinal mass
    D. Complaints of left flank pain

Rationale:

Correct answer: C

Non-Hodgkin's lymphoma is cancer that begins in lymphocytes. A mediastinal mass should be ruled out in patients newly diagnosed with the cancer as this can progress to respiratory distress, tracheal compression, and superior vena cava syndrome, which is a medical emergency.

A is incorrect because white blood cell counts in non-Hodgkin's lymphoma is usually decreased.

B is incorrect because the uric acid level is normal.

D is incorrect because complaints of left flank pain is important to assess but is not as urgent as a mediastinal mass.

15. The nurse on the pediatric oncology unit is administering vincristine sulfate to a 5-year-old boy with a brain stem glioma. Which of the following adverse reactions does the nurse monitor for?

    A. Typhlitis
    B. Diarrhea
    C. Constipation
    D. Appendicitis

Rationale:

Correct answer: C

A brain stem glioma is either a benign or malignant collection of cells that form in brain tissue. Vincristine sulfate is vinka alkaloid antineoplastic medication which works by inhibiting cancerous cell division. It is used to treat Hodgkin's disease and other lymphomas and cancers. Side effects include neuropathy, such as in the intestines, which can lead to constipation. It is also a priority to assess the IV site regularly because infiltration of this medication can be very toxic to the surrounding tissues.

A is incorrect because typhlitis (an infectious process that can arise during neutropenic episodes) is not common with vinka alkaloid medication administration.

B is incorrect because constipation is more likely to occur with vinka alkaloid medications.

D is incorrect because appendicitis is an infectious process that can arise during neutropenic episodes, not related to vinka alkaloid administration.

Multiple Response

16. The nurse on the pediatric oncology unit is caring for a 10-year-old girl with a brain tumor. Which of the following observations would the nurse report immediately to the healthcare provider? (Select all that apply.)

    A. Urine output decrease from 40 ml/hr. to 25 ml/hr.
    B. Vomiting
    C. Visual changes
    D. Abdominal discomfort
    E. Diarrhea
    F. Headache

Rationale:

Correct answer: B, C, F

Vomiting, visual changes, and headache are all clinical manifestations of space occupying intracranial lesions or ventriculo-peritoneal shunt malfunction. These symptoms should be reported to the healthcare provider immediately.

A is incorrect because slightly decreased urine output does not require immediate reporting. This is still a normal urine output for a 10-year-old patient.

D is incorrect because abdominal discomfort requires further assessment but does not require immediate reporting to the healthcare provider.

E is incorrect because diarrhea may be a side effect of medications and does not require immediate reporting to the healthcare provider until the nurse assesses further.

17. The nurse is planning care for a 6-year-old male patient with hemophilia who requires factor VIII replacement twice weekly. Which of the following does the nurse include in the plan of care? (Select all that apply.)

    A. Avoid IV puncture due to risk of bleeding
    B. Maintain bedrest if acute bleeding occurs
    C. Take rectal temperature every 4 hours and report fever to healthcare provider
    D. Administer low-dose aspirin for pain instead of narcotics
    E. Avoid intramuscular injections

Rationale:

Correct answer: B, E

Hemophilia is a hereditary blood disorder in which the patent experiences lack of coagulation factors, which severely reduces the clotting ability of the blood. If the patient begins acutely bleeding, strict bedrest must be maintained. Intramuscular injections are not generally needed during treatment for hemophilia and should be avoided due to the risk for bleeding.

A is incorrect because IV access is necessary in order to administer factor VIII replacement. The nurse should monitor the IV site frequently for bleeding.

C is incorrect because rectal procedures and suppositories should be avoided in patients with hemophilia due to the risk for bleeding due to reduced ability of the blood to clot.

D is incorrect because salicylate medications, such as aspirin, increase the risk for bleeding and are inappropriate for a 6-year-old patient.

18. The nurse is providing teaching to the parents of a 7-year-old boy with phenylketonuria (PKU). Which of the statements by the parents indicates the teaching is understood? (Select all that apply.)

    A. "He will essentially be a vegetarian because he cannot have meat products."
    B. "He must avoid all types of bread and pasta."
    C. "No fresh flowers in his room."
    D. "Diet ginger ale is acceptable in small quantities to help with nausea."
    E. "Oher than the Guthrie test done at birth, no other routine blood testing will be necessary."
    F. "He will have to learn to keep a food diary."

Rationale:

Correct answer: A, F

Phenylketonuria (PKU) is an inborn error of phenylalanine metabolism due to deficiency of a specific liver enzyme. Toxic metabolites can build up in the blood, leading to brain cell death and subsequent intellectual delay, seizures, and mental disorders. Foods that must be avoided include meat, eggs, and dairy products. A food diary must be kept in order to monitor the amount of phenylalanine the patient consumes daily. Food exchange lists (similar to those for patients with diabetes) can help the patient with swapping foods, depending on different choices made throughout the day.

B is incorrect because specially made low-protein breads and pastas are available for PKU patients, so they can still consume these foods in controlled quantities.

C is incorrect because PKU patients are not at specific risk for infection while hospitalized, and thus, fresh flowers are acceptable in the room.

D is incorrect because aspartame, used to sweeten diet soda, contains large amounts of phenylalanine and can be harmful. If the child is going to drink sweetened beverages, those sweetened with sugar are safer than diet options.

E is incorrect because routine bloodwork may be necessary to monitor phenylalanine levels in the blood.

19. The new nurse in the pediatric unit is caring for a male 4-year-old child with Duchenne Muscular Dystrophy (DMD). Which of the following statements is appropriate for the nurse to make when educating the child's parents? (Select all that apply.)

    A. "This disorder may have resulted from lack of oxygen at birth."

A. “Your child may be at increased risk for eczema.”
B. “It is important to call the healthcare provider if you observe any signs of seizure activity.”
C. “PKU increases the risk for developing Attention Deficit Disorder (ADD).”
D. “You may notice more impulsive behavior in your child due to the effects of PKU on the brain.”
E. “Motor problems may occur. Additional therapy is available to help your child develop fine and gross motor skills.”

Rationale:

Correct answer: A, B, D, E

Phenylketonuria (PKU) is a recessive gene disorder that causes the liver to not produce enzymes to break down phenylalanine (amino acid), which then accumulates and is toxic to the brain. Children with PKU are at risk for developing eczema, seizures, impulsiveness, and motor problems.

C is incorrect because ADD is not a risk related to PKU.

22. The nurse in the pediatric emergency room is caring for a 9-year-old girl in sickle cell crisis. Her hemoglobin is 10 g/dL, and she is complaining of severe pain in her leg joints. Which of the following does the nurse anticipate implementing? (Select all that apply.)

A. Folic acid supplements
B. High-iron foods
C. Ice packs to leg joints
D. IV fluids
E. IV morphine

Rationale:

Correct answer: A, D, E

Sickle cell disease is a hereditary anemia which mutates hemoglobin and distorts red blood cells to a sickle or crescent shape when oxygen levels are low. In order to manage the sickle cell crisis, the nurse anticipates folic acid supplements for erythropoiesis, IV fluids to decrease blood viscosity, and IV morphine for pain control.

B is incorrect because high-iron foods are not necessary for sickle cell crisis.

C is incorrect because ice packs would cause further sickling of red blood cells.

23. The nurse is providing dietary teaching to the parents of a 6-year-old recently diagnosed with phenylketonuria (PKU). Which of the following dietary choices indicate the teaching has been successful? (Select all that apply.)

    A. Bananas with peanut butter
    B. Green beans with olive oil and salt
    C. Chicken with potatoes
    D. Turkey and steamed carrots
    E. Sugar-based lollipop

Rationale:

Correct answer: B, E

Phenylketonuria (PKU) is a recessive gene disorder that causes the liver to not produce enzymes to break down phenylalanine (amino acid), which then accumulates and is toxic to the brain. Dietary choices for children with PKU include fruits, vegetables, and low-protein natural foods. Sugar-based candies that do not contain protein, dairy, or aspartame (artificial sweetener) are acceptable treats.

A is incorrect because, although a banana is a good choice for a PKU patient, the peanut butter is high in protein.

C is incorrect because chicken is high in protein.

D is incorrect because turkey is high in protein.

24. The nurse in the pediatric intensive care unit (PICU) is caring for a 7-year-old girl after a craniotomy surgery for removal of a brain tumor. When assessing the child, for which of the following should the nurse notify the healthcare provider? (Select all that apply.)

    A. Absence of pronator drift
    B. The patient frequently requests water to drink
    C. Polyuria
    D. Pupils react slowly to light accommodation
    E. Blood pressure changes from 95/65 to 118/58

Rationale:

Correct answer: C, D, E

Polyuria can be a manifestation of diabetes insipidus, a complication after craniotomy. Pupils should respond quickly light; sluggish pupil reaction can be an early sign of increasing intracranial pressure (ICP). Increased pulse pressure is a sign of increasing ICP and should be reported to the healthcare provider. (Note: Pulse pressure is the difference between the systolic and diastolic pressure and is normally 30-40 mm/Hg.)

A is incorrect because absence of pronator drift is a good finding post-craniotomy. Pronator drift can be an indication of increasing intracranial pressure.

B is incorrect because thirst is common post-operatively and is not a sign of a complication.

25. A 9-year-old boy is hospitalized for leukemia and receiving combination chemotherapy. Lab results indicate neutropenia, and the nurse is preparing to implement protective isolation. Which of the following interventions does the nurse initiate? (Select all that apply.)

A. Restrict all visitors
B. Place on a low-bacteria diet
C. Delegate the nursing assistant to change dressings using sterile technique
D. Encourage fresh fruits and vegetables
E. Meticulous handwashing before care
F. Fresh-cut flowers allowed if vase water is changed daily

Rationale:

Correct answer: B, E

Leukemia is a malignant disease which causes increased numbers of abnormal or immature leukocytes to be produced from the bone marrow and blood-forming organs, suppressing normal blood cell production. Vegetables and fruits can harbor microorganisms which can lead to infections in the immunocompromised child. All fruits and vegetables should be peeled or cooked. Dressing changes should be performed using sterile technique. Meticulous handwashing is priority for the neutropenic child.

A is incorrect because not all visitors should be restricted, only those who are ill.

C is incorrect. Although a sterile technique is needed for all dressing changes for a patient on neutropenic precautions, the nurse cannot delegate sterile procedures to the nursing assistant.

D is incorrect because fresh fruits and vegetables can harbor microorganisms, increasing the risk for infection.

F is incorrect because standing water in a vase, even when changed daily, can harbor microorganisms.

Made in the USA
Las Vegas, NV
19 October 2023

79332227R00103